Careers in Medicine, Dentistry and Mental Health

SEVENTH EDITION

JUDITH HUMPHRIES
AND LOULOU BROWN

KOGAN PAGE
CAREERS SERIES

First published in 1981
Second edition 1985
Third edition 1988
Fourth edition 1989
Fifth edition 1992
Sixth edition 1994
Seventh edition 1996

Kogan Page Limited
120 Pentonville Road
London N1 9JN

British Library Cataloguing in Publication Data
A CIP record for this book is available from the British Library.
ISBN 0-7494-1783-8

Typeset by Kogan Page
Printed and bound in Great Britain by Clays Ltd, St Ives plc

Contents

Introduction 5

1. **Basic Medical Training** 9
Applying for a Course 9; Course Structure 10; Life as a Medical Student 11; Grants and Loans 11; The Pre-registration Year 11; Conditions of Work 13; Qualities Required 14; Finding a Pre-registration Post 14; Registration 14

2. **The Hospital Doctor** 15
Working for the National Health Service 15; Training 15; Specialties 16; Surgery 18; Medicine 19; Pathology 20; Anaesthetics, Radiology and Radiotherapy 22; Obstetrics and Gynaecology 23; Becoming a Consultant 23; Salary Scales 24; Finding a Job 24

3. **The Doctor in the Community** 25
Introduction 25; General Practice 25; Community Health 29; Public Health Medicine 30

4. **Dentistry** 33
Introduction 33; Training 33; Registration 34; General Practice 34; Working in a Hospital 37; Orthodontics 37; Oral Surgery 38; The Community Dental Service 38; Occupational and Industrial Practice 40; Salary Scales 41; Finding a Job 41

5. **Working for the Armed Services and Working Abroad** 42
The Armed Services 42; Working Abroad 45

6. **Complementary and Alternative Medicine** 49
Introduction 49; Qualities Required of Practitioners 49; The Status of Complementary Medicine 50; Organisation of Training and Practice 50; Natural Therapies 50; Acupuncture 51; Alexander Technique 52; Healing 53;

Herbal Medicine 54; Homoeopathy 54; Hypnotherapy 55; Osteopathy 55

7. Mental Health **57**
Introduction 57; Work Settings 58; Training and Professional Functions 58; Working in Hospitals 59; Working in the Community 61; Salary Scales 63; Finding a Job 63

8. Professional Qualifications and Training Courses **64**
Medical and Dental Undergraduate Courses 64; Higher Medical and Dental Qualifications 68; Postgraduate Awards 68; Courses in Complementary Medicine 82; Professional Training in Mental Health 85

9. Useful Addresses **92**
General 92; Medical 92; Dentistry 94; Complementary Medicine 95; Mental Health 96

Introduction

This book draws together career opportunities across the whole field of health care. It is intended for people whose educational background equips them to take a course which will qualify them to practise independently – for instance as a doctor, dentist, psychologist or osteopath. In general, this means that you must fulfil the requirements for university entrance and, particularly for entry to medical and dental schools, be reasonably confident of getting good A-level results. It also means that you must be willing to spend a considerable number of years in training, as a period of postgraduate study or training is a normal requirement in most cases.

Both the undergraduate and postgraduate aspects of training are dealt with and, for this reason, the information should be useful both to sixth-formers and to students who are making decisions about their future careers. Because the choice is wide these decisions can be difficult, so we have attempted to identify the main factors influencing choice and relate them to the actual experience of people working in various settings and disciplines. This is done through a series of case studies, which are conversations with people who were chosen because they represent a wide spectrum of interests and opinions. The views expressed may not necessarily be our own, but they serve to give a picture of the diversity of opportunities available. This book does not outline many jobs below graduate level. Details of job opportunities in the Health Service for school leavers are available in other Kogan Page titles, such as *Careers in Nursing and Related Professions* by Linda Nazarko.

Medicine. Much of the book is about doctors: how to become one and then how to decide what kind of doctor you want to be. The training structure is complex and, although explanatory literature is available to all medical students, this is very factual in its approach and not always helpful with the problems of actually making a choice. Personal accounts in the form of case studies seem more relevant. What are the rewards and pressures, both of training and of subsequent practice? Where do people feel they have made mistakes? What considerations are uppermost when people decide to work in one area rather than another?

Years ago, medicine was thought of as a male preserve, and to some extent this attitude still survives. For this reason, it is important that women should know what their position within the profession is likely to be in advance. Although there is now no barrier to women becoming students, the system, particularly as regards postgraduate training, is in fact discriminatory, in that it takes no account of possible family commitments. Within hospitals, women predominate in the 'unpopular' specialties. These also tend to be the ones concerned with personal and social problems rather than with highly technological treatment procedures, so whether women on the whole tend to be temperamentally more attracted to this kind of work, or settle for it because it is accessible to them, is an open question. But it cannot be denied that, in a competitive field with little provision for the part-time jobs women often need, there is still little incentive to create part-time posts in popular areas where plenty of full-time applicants are available.

Dentistry. Dentistry is, on the whole, less of a competitive jungle than medicine, and has the advantage of a shorter training period. Career opportunities are not as diverse as they are in medicine, but general practice, where most dentists are employed, offers a very independent working situation. Although you will be bound, to some extent, by financial considerations, you will have the freedom to develop your own ideas and style of working and – an important consideration for women – be able to set your own working hours.

Complementary and Alternative Medicine. Complementary and alternative medicine describes treatment given through therapies such as osteopathy and acupuncture which operate without recourse to pharmacological drugs. There are many such therapies in existence and to practise them you will need the technical skill particular to each one and some degree of background medical knowledge, depending on the subject area. The important common feature in all forms of complementary and alternative medicine is that treatment is given holistically, that is, with regard to the whole person. You have to be in sympathy with this method of treating illness if you are going to work in this field.

Mental Health. Mental health care is the meeting point of the Health, Social, and Education Services and people can come to this work via any of these disciplines. The very fact that it demands an all-round view of the patient is its attraction for many people. New moves to create more provision at the early stages of illness are gradually leading to the growth of interesting jobs, within the community as well as in the more traditional hospital settings. It is as well to note, however, that training is a lengthy process in this field, as a first degree must be followed by relevant work experience and a course of professional training.

The first aim of all people with a responsibility for any form of health care must be to improve the well-being of their patients, but there are many opinions as to how this is best achieved. Frequently there are changes in emphasis, both in actual methods of treatment and in the organisation of the services providing it. New research gives rise to new approaches. Some of the issues currently involved are discussed, along with descriptions of the work areas. Everyone involved in medicine will need to have a strong, personal ideology for the basis of his or her work if it is to extend beyond the technical limits of professional expertise and also become an appropriate personal and social service.

The publishers would like to thank all those who took the trouble to answer their letters, supply information and comment on the text. Wherever possible, we have used information coming from primary sources, ie from professional organisations, examining bodies and those working in the field. When we received no satisfactory reply to our requests for information we were forced to turn to secondary sources.

Chapter 1

Basic Medical Training

Applying for a Course

There are 27 medical schools in the UK, eight of which are in London. Each is attached both to a university and to a hospital or hospital group. Applicants are usually required to be between the ages of 18 and 30 at the time their studies begin, and at some medical schools the upper age limit can be as low as 25. Competition for medical school places is very keen, with deans usually giving priority to school leavers starting their first university courses. Very few places are therefore available for mature students. Official entry requirements are three A levels at either grade A or grade B in chemistry and other science subjects, although there are some opportunities for people who have not taken the right subjects at A level, but who are otherwise academically well qualified, to take a first MB course in basic science subjects. This will qualify them to apply for further medical training, but these courses are few and far between. Graduate candidates normally require a first or upper second class honours degree.

The traditional bias against women has been disclaimed and schools are now, on principle, prepared to accept equal numbers of both sexes, though the extent to which this actually happens will vary from place to place and according to the balance of demand. Several women we spoke to who had recently finished their training in medicine or dentistry said they felt that they had to do better than the men in order that their work should gain recognition. There does still seem to be a tendency for schools to recruit a large number of students from families with medical backgrounds, and some schools will only take applicants who make them their first choice. This, again, will vary and the best method of finding out the score for individual schools is by personal enquiry.

Scottish applicants to Scottish medical schools are accepted on their results in their SCEs. After taking SCEs applicants are generally required to study for an additional year and to pass the Scottish Certificate of Sixth Year Studies. There is no evidence that medical schools will take any previous degrees or work experience into consideration. People we spoke to felt that age probably went against them and that they were still judged by the same academic criteria as school leavers.

Details of application procedures are given in Chapter 8.

Course Structure

The basic medical course lasts for five years and can last for six years for students who take an extra year to qualify for a BSc (at Cambridge a BA) in Medical Sciences, or for those who insert an intercalated degree course.

The course is divided into two parts: the second MB or pre-clinical period, and the clinical period. For the first two years students learn basic medical sciences. Studies during this time include pathology, physiology, pharmacology, biochemistry and anatomy (which involves dissection of the human body). Some medical schools teach psychology and medical sociology as ancillary subjects. For this part of the course, students will work the ordinary university terms and the work will be mainly lecture and laboratory based.

The course is beset with exams. By the end of the second year students should have passed their second MB examination. At this point most universities encourage students of ability to 'intercalate' an extra year studying a single basic medical subject to honours degree level. At Oxford and Cambridge the intercalated year is compulsory. Most students carry straight on to the last three years, during which sickness and disease are dealt with. The period is spent mainly in teaching hospitals and involves observation of patients and of the doctors dealing with them. The field of studies is wide and includes clinical method, which is the study of finding out information about patients and their illnesses; pathology, which is the academic study of disease; and the application of these two studies to the various specialties. These are the specialist areas of medical and surgical knowledge and practice from which, eventually, each student will have to choose in deciding on a career.

Experience comes from attachment to 'firms', or medical teams, for eight- to ten-week periods. Some firms are general medicine or surgery; others are more specialised. Students move from firm to firm during the three clinical years and the course is backed up by lectures, demonstrations and discussions. They become familiar with working in hospital wards, get their first introduction to patients and learn the techniques of making physical examinations and obtaining the patients' medical histories. The role assigned to students within the hospital is very humble. They will have a lot of routine tasks to perform, will find themselves being deferential to members of staff, and may generally feel unappreciated. There is also a two-month period in the final year, known as the 'elective', which may be spent, within reason, as each student chooses. Many people take this as an opportunity to go abroad and experience medical work in a Third World country. Others may choose to contribute to a research project. Grants are not generally available, but most medical schools have some sources of funding to help students who wish to go abroad.

During the clinical years, students are expected to work for periods in a full hospital schedule, including some night duties, and will have four weeks' holiday each year. At the end of the three years the final examinations are taken. These are qualifying examinations but do not yet confer the right to practise. This right is only conferred by registration with the General Medical Council after a further pre-registration year of hospital work.

Life as a Medical Student

Medical students can find themselves isolated from other people, although this may be less of a problem in medical schools attached to universities. Medical schools tend not to have the range of societies and social groups to be found in the wider setting of a university and for some people this can be limiting. (One person we spoke to described social life at her medical school as being composed of rugger, beer and Christian Union!) The pressure of work is greater, creating the need to concentrate almost entirely on the prescribed area of study, and students have little or no time to indulge in more general intellectual exploration and exchange of ideas. On the bonus side, however, the work is interesting, teaching in most medical schools is of a high standard, and there is the satisfying feeling of pursuing a clear objective.

Grants and Loans

Medical courses are expensive but most students who have not previously taken a first degree course should be able to obtain a grant from their local education authority. Mature students who already have a first degree are likely to face considerable financial problems as local education authorities have no obligation to support students on further degree courses. Medical schools increasingly insist on a financial guarantee before considering mature candidates. Student loans are available to bridge the gap between grants and expenditure. (For details consult the Educational Grants Advisory Service or the British Medical Association Education Trust – see p. 92.)

During the clinical years when students must support themselves for longer than the usual 30 weeks of university terms, additional allowances are made. Most medical schools have various scholarships for which there is open competition. These do not usually amount to much money, but they can be a help, or enable a student to finance a special project. Applications for LEA grants are made to the 'home' authority in the year prior to becoming a student.

The Pre-registration Year

After qualifying, all doctors' paths are the same for one year. They must work under supervision as a house officer in general hospitals. At this time they have a salary and a set role in the hierarchy of hospital life. When they have completed this year satisfactorily, they can be fully registered with the General Medical Council. No examinations are involved.

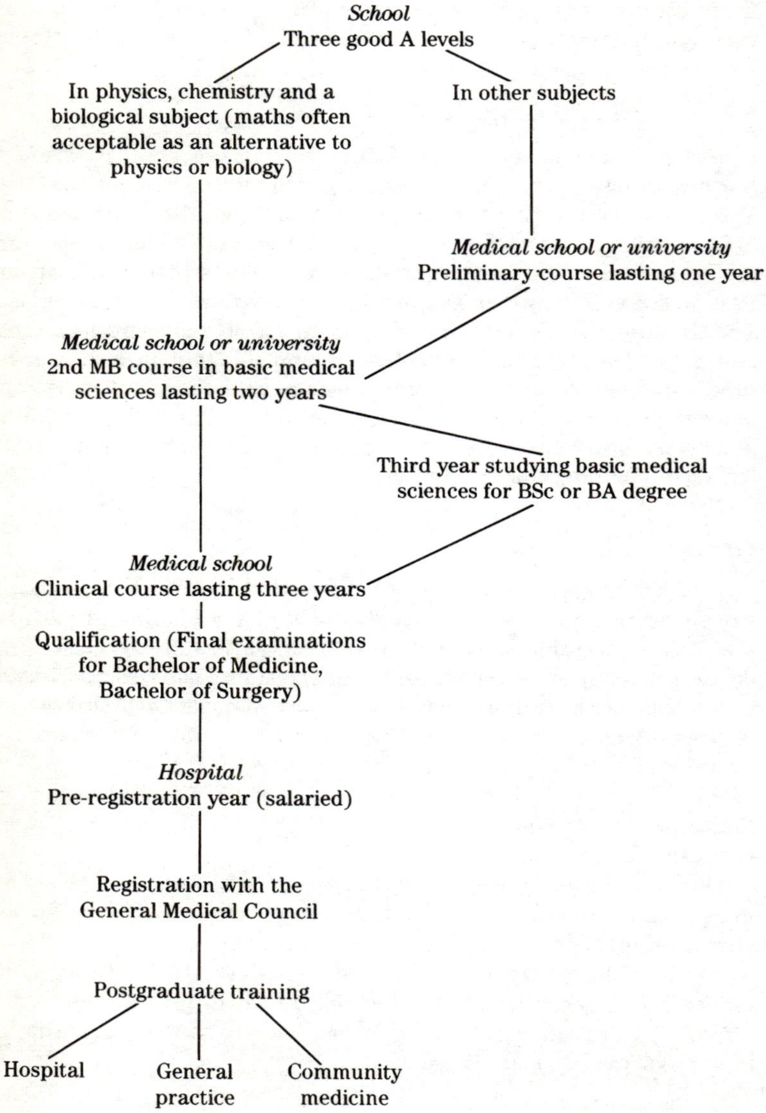

Figure 1. *Training routes to registration and subsequent career choices*

The pre-registration year is usually divided between two six-month posts, one as house physician and one as house surgeon. This should give the young doctor a considerable range of experience from which to make the necessary choices for a future career.

Conditions of Work

Life as a house officer is hard. In spite of concerns raised by junior doctors and the Department of Health's agreement to limit the hours worked by junior doctors to no more than 72 hours per week, it is very likely that for the foreseeable future junior doctors will often be working up to, or sometimes in excess of, 80 hours per week. The reduction in hours is being phased in over the next few years. It is also important to note that there are long periods of 'on call' duties, especially at nights and over weekends. Hospital work has become more acute over the last ten years. In the past, junior doctors spent a lot of 'on call' time sleeping or relaxing; this, however, has changed.

Although much of the work will be interesting and rewarding, there is a good deal of routine clerical work to be got through, and you will generally be the person on hand for the more run-of-the-mill tasks. You will get four weeks' holiday a year and your salary will range from £13,930 to £15,730 (1995), with extra payments for out-of-hours work.

Case Study

A young doctor remembers his pre-registration year as a House Officer

> It's hard work and very demanding, but it feels good to be doing something useful after being a student and feeling rather superfluous. Having a recognised role is nice, too. The actual work entails being in the hospital from nine until six each day, with one half-day off each week. In addition you are on call every third night and third weekend. This might mean just watching television and waiting for something to happen, or it might mean working all night. The weekends are the worst – by Sunday evening you feel pretty awful.
>
> I worked on just one or two wards and had the care of a group of about 20 to 30 patients. This meant seeing them every day, monitoring their progress and talking to them and their relatives – you are the person who has the time for this, though not always enough of it. Otherwise, your time is spent chasing up investigations and getting ready for the week's high spot – the consultant's ward round. I found the day-to-day contact with the patients satisfying and working on the same wards you get to know the staff well, so the relationships can be quite good.
>
> Sometimes you feel like a dogsbody. There's a lot of clerical work, form filling in and so forth, and chasing around, especially in a large teaching hospital.
>
> In my medical post I also worked in outpatient clinics, and while working in surgery I assisted at operations. Often this means long hours on one's feet in the theatre when all you might be doing is holding back pieces of skin so that the consultant can operate. That's very tiring. But I did get to do a few minor operations – removing bumps, appendixes and so forth, and I found that satisfying. I think the pay is reasonable – especially as you have no time to spend it except during your four weeks' holiday!

Qualities Required

Being a medical student is physically, intellectually and emotionally demanding. During your studies you will have to absorb an enormous volume of knowledge, and work long hours in physically demanding conditions. As soon as you qualify you will be thrown in at the deep end as far as human relationships are concerned. You will have seen from the case study that the young hospital doctor has the primary personal contact with patients. This means that you will often be required to sort out patients' problems and fears about their illnesses, as well as dealing with worried relatives. You will have to present a confident and reassuring manner while still remaining in a subordinate position in the hospital hierarchy.

The length of training involved should not be underestimated. After the six or seven years described in this chapter, which brings most people well into their mid-20s, doctors must still pursue further postgraduate training before they can become fully independent in their chosen branch of medicine.

Finding a Pre-registration Post

Although the pre-registration year is part of the basic medical training process, allocation to a post is not automatic. Most medical schools operate a 'matching plan' similar to that used by UCAS, by which the wishes of graduates and the needs of consultants are matched as far as possible. But difficulties can arise if you want to gain experience in an unusual sphere.

Most approved pre-registration posts are in general or district hospitals in the area in which the medical school is situated. It is not possible to obtain a post at a specialist hospital as they do not usually employ doctors in house officer grades.

In each medical school there will be a staff member who has the responsibility for organising allocation to pre-registration posts.

Registration

If you wish to qualify as a doctor in the UK, you must first obtain, by examination, a primary qualification which confers a title to registration under the Medical Act. You are then entitled to apply for provisional registration, and after satisfactorily completing one year as a student house officer in approved hospitals, you are eligible to apply for full registration. The General Medical Council keeps the Register of all qualified medical practitioners. For details of primary qualifications see *British Qualifications* (Kogan Page), published annually.

Chapter 2

The Hospital Doctor

Working for the National Health Service

Roughly 25 per cent of doctors work in hospitals and more than 95 per cent of newly graduated doctors begin their careers working in a hospital within the National Health Service (NHS). Although some NHS hospitals take private patients, it is up to individual doctors (usually, only at consultant level) to decide whether they are willing to take on private work. Working for the Health Service is, therefore, the norm and is described in this chapter.

Training

Training Posts

The first four grades of hospital medical staff are known as training posts. These are house officer, senior house officer, registrar and senior registrar. They represent a set hierarchy of responsibility and, while moving through them, all doctors work under the supervision of the consultant who also has responsibility for their postgraduate training. The atmosphere is very competitive, each post being held for a specified time after which the doctor must seek another. It is only at consultant level that doctors are considered to be fully trained and fully independent. Staff grade doctors and associated specialists have permanent appointments but are not fully independent.

Postgraduate Training

While working in training posts, doctors combine their working life with postgraduate study and further examinations. Doctors move around the various specialties in posts of six or twelve months' duration, and must maintain a demanding working pace. This will decline somewhat in the higher grades but the pressures of work and examinations will continue to be high for some time.

Postgraduate training is rather in the nature of an apprenticeship. All hospital doctors eventually work in a specialty which they learn on the job with the aid of any optional short courses which may be available. Higher examinations are a necessity for promotion. These are not university degrees but professional awards of the Royal Colleges of the various specialties. Most are taken in two parts and all have a written and practical component. The pass rate of these examinations is very low, sometimes only 10 to 15 per cent. It is therefore common for exams to be taken more than once.

The general pattern of postgraduate training consists of about three years of general training in areas relevant to the eventual specialty, followed by four years of specialist training, usually in senior registrar posts. Sometimes, both parts of the examination of the Royal College concerned are taken during the general training period and act as a qualification for admission to specialist training. Sometimes it is possible to take Part 2 of the examination after embarking on specialist training.

Part-time Training

The British Medical Association (BMA) is anxious to promote part-time training, and since 1990 5 per cent of whole-time equivalent registrar posts have been reserved for part-time training. The Department of Health has acknowledged that opportunities for part-time posts are inadequate at present. The BMA has set up a working party on doctors which has considered the hours of work and their effect on family life.

The demands of the postgraduate training period can be particularly difficult for some women who may have commitments to young children during this time. Opportunities for part-time training are limited and depend largely on the exercising of personal initiative. Hospital doctors in training can apply to job-share a full-time establishment post, or a part-time post, but for this they will need the approval of the relevant Royal College and the funding authority. Details of these part-time training schemes are available from postgraduate deans, clinical tutors and employing authorities. For those who are unable to work at least half-time, there is the doctors' retainer scheme which allows doctors to work a maximum of one day a week and attend a minimum of seven educational sessions a year. The Medical Women's Federation (MWF), Tavistock House North, Tavistock Square, London WC1H 9HX has a network of careers advisers throughout the UK who can provide information, advice and counselling for members wishing to work either full- or part-time. The MWF also publishes a journal *Medical Woman* which from time to time carries articles on careers, including part-time opportunities, in different specialties.

Specialties

The tendency towards specialisation is increasing all the time. It is impossible to list the innumerable specialties and sub-specialties within hospital work. For practical purposes, however, these can be divided into groups which can be aligned with the various colleges: surgery, medicine, pathology, psychiatry, anaesthetics, radiology, obstetrics and gynaecology. Apart from psychiatry, which is dealt with in Chapter 7, this chapter is concerned with all specialties mentioned.

Although there are areas of overlap where people from one discipline work in co-operation with those from another, these groups of specialties are quite clearly defined, not only in terms of the interests and skills they require but also in terms of the personalities and temperaments of the people they are likely to attract. The responsibilities and rewards of each are very different and many people, while still undergraduates, will find themselves drawn to one area more than another.

Choosing a Specialty

Newly qualified doctors are well advised to choose their specialty early in their working life, and obviously their choice will depend not only on their personal interests but also on the general conditions of work and career

Medicine	
Audiological medicine	General medicine
Cardiology	Geriatric medicine
Clinical genetics	Infectious diseases
Clinical neurophysiology	Medical oncology
Clinical pharmacology and therapeutics	Nephrology
	Neurology
Clinical physiology	Nuclear medicine
Dermatology	Paediatrics
Diseases of the chest	Rheumatology
Endocrinology	Venereology
Gastroenterology	
Pathology	
Blood transfusion	Histopathology
Chemical pathology	Immunopathology
General pathology	Microbiology
Haematology	Neuropathology
Psychiatry	
Child and adolescent psychiatry	Mental handicap
Forensic psychiatry	Mental illness (adult)
Psychotherapy	
Surgery	
Accident and emergency	Ophthalmology
Cardiothoracic surgery	Paediatric surgery
Ear, nose and throat	Plastic surgery
General surgery	Traumatic and orthopaedic surgery
Neurosurgery	Urology
Other	
Anaesthetics	Radiology
Gynaecology and obstetrics	Radiotherapy

Table 1. *Main hospital specialties*

prospects. The main factor influencing working conditions is the nature of the illness being dealt with and the likely incidence of emergency cases. Someone working in orthopaedic surgery (that is, dealing with broken and injured bones), for instance, is likely to have far more out-of-hours work than a dermatologist, who treats skin diseases. Both will have their set times of night and weekend duty but the working pace this entails will usually be quite different.

Women doctors are more heavily concentrated in less 'acute' specialties, such as radiology, anaesthetics or geriatrics because 'on call' commitment (that is, the time spent either at home or in the hospital awaiting emergencies) is less. This allows them to combine a position of responsibility with bringing up children.

There is, equally, a great disparity in the career prospects of different specialties. There are popular and unpopular ones; the ones which have a high growth rate and those which do not. In general, surgical specialties have a low growth rate and correspondingly high competition for jobs. Most medical specialties are popular and therefore relatively difficult to get into, but career prospects in geriatric medicine, dermatology and medical audiology are good. Pathology, the study of disease, also offers good career prospects.

Surgery

Surgery is concerned with patients who need operations. Surgeons tend to have a practical view of illness. Their task is specific – they must use their skill in a very tangible way to solve a particular problem. Often their interest is restricted to that aspect of the patient for which the operation is required and this may well be at the expense of an all-round view of the patient as a person. Some distancing of this kind may be necessary in surgery where unpleasant mutilations may have to be performed and there are always some patients who die as a result of the surgeon's work.

On the other hand, the surgeon will assume complete responsibility for each patient both before, during and after the operation. In no other branch of medicine is one person so directly responsible for the outcome of the treatment given.

Case Study

A talk with a Consultant General Surgeon

> Surgery is very satisfying – I feel immensely privileged being able to do it. I have a pride in being a craftsman and using my skill in a useful way. I like the independent working situation, the personal responsibility. I would not do a major operation if I was unable to follow up on the subsequent progress of the patient. Not many of us are keen on the team concept of working, though that obviously comes into it to some extent.
>
> As a surgeon, you have to get used to the fact of death. I think this is why surgeons tend to be a bit extrovert, with not too much insight. Too much

soul-searching is bad for the patient and for you. Surgery is not, on the whole, a terribly intellectual pursuit. If you have difficult diagnostic problems you can ask a physician for help. This means that you can keep on doing it. There are not the problems of keeping up with the younger people that there are in other areas. I do most of my 'keeping up' through conferences and meetings which I find more useful than reading.

I think it's a pity that the present training structure seems to be keeping women out of surgery. It is not practically possible to have part-time posts in surgery because of the personal commitment to patients, and many women during the training period can only work part time. What we need is an alternative training scheme beginning at the age of 35 or so, but I doubt that would be acceptable on economic grounds.

Medicine

Medicine is concerned with caring for patients who do not need operations. Although there are many routine methods of investigation and treatment, the task of the physician can often be less specific than that of the surgeon. Where there is an element of doubt, doctors must rely to a large extent on their personal judgement both for interpreting the available information and in deciding treatment. This is a challenge which makes medicine attractive to many people.

There are many different specialties within medicine. Some deal with patients who have acute illnesses, for whom it is usually possible to suggest some fairly well-defined curative treatment. Others deal with people who have long-term disorders and need periodic hospital care for the management of their illnesses. In these cases, there is a lasting commitment to the patient who may never, in any sense, be 'cured'. In all situations, doctors work in a team and can rely on specialist help from colleagues in other disciplines where appropriate.

Paediatrics

Paediatrics is general medicine as applied to children. It covers the whole age range from the neo-natal period up to puberty, and sometimes beyond. In hospitals, doctors are dealing only with new-born or sick children but they also need to know about the development of healthy children and the facilities available to them in the community. For this reason it is a good idea, during the training period, to get away from the hospital for a time and work in a child health clinic or development assessment centre.

One of the special features of paediatrics is that the patients often cannot tell you what is wrong. Young children, particularly, are very much a diagnostic challenge, and communication must be through the parents or the adults close to them.

In paediatrics, the working pace is varied and unpredictable and there is likely to be much out-of-hours work. Nevertheless, it is a popular specialty, and competition for jobs is high.

Case Study

A Paediatrician outlines her work

When I was working in surgery as a house officer, I disliked the time spent waiting for the patients to be anaesthetised and, anyway, I found the diagnostic challenge of medical patients much more rewarding than being a technician, just operating. Originally I thought of doing medicine as a preparation for specialising in pathology, but as a student I did my pathology after I'd done some paediatrics and I found I missed the children. At that point I decided to become a paediatrician.

I didn't know if I could cope, emotionally, with very sick children, so I went to a post at the Hospital for Sick Children at Great Ormond Street. Very few children actually die in district hospitals, whereas at Great Ormond Street there can be as many as 500 deaths a year, so this was a good test. Once I was involved, I didn't find this a burden at all. Of course, I got very upset – I still do – when children died. But often, sadly, these deaths can be a relief after long and difficult illnesses. It is only the occasional ones involving previously healthy children or accident cases which are really difficult to accept.

After my pre-registration year, I did three senior house officer jobs, one in general medicine and the others in obstetrics and gynaecology, and neonatology. Then I had a two-year period as a registrar which was divided between two posts, one at a general hospital and the other at a teaching hospital, when I did general paediatrics and more neonatology. After this I got my present job, and spent the first two years of it doing research. I think research is an important part of training as it can take you out of the hospital or into allied areas such as obstetrics and gynaecology and child psychiatry, and give you a broader view.

I like the atmosphere of paediatric wards. Children are much nicer as patients, and when they are better they will let you know. They have no self-awareness to hinder their recovery. They don't think of themselves as sick or feel sorry for themselves. In fact, they have a much greater pain tolerance than adults but lose this as they grow up. They are much happier too – paediatric wards are always noisier and more chaotic than others, and very friendly places.

It *can* be hard work, though. Children, and particularly babies, don't respect the time of day or night. Technically, too, you must be very skilled. You are working on a smaller scale and you can't be clumsy. But the atmosphere on the wards and the fact that you are working, not with patients as individuals but with the whole family, makes this a very special job for me.

Pathology

Pathology is the study of disease, of its causation and its effect on the body. Pathologists help clinicians with diagnosis and can also be involved with making recommendations for treatment and assessing the subsequent progress of patients. Most of the work is laboratory based and, though there can be some contact with patients, this is usually in an advisory capacity and in co-operation with the doctors treating them.

There is a whole range of laboratory techniques used in pathology and these fall under four main groupings:

Chemical Pathology. This involves the measurement of chemical substances in the body, such as salts, hormones etc. The pathologist's job is to decide which tests are most appropriate in individual cases and to interpret the results in the light of knowledge obtained about the patient.

Haematology. This is the study of blood. The haematologist measures such things as the number and character of blood cells, and is also concerned with bone marrow which is involved in the production of blood. Of all branches of pathology, haematology affords the most contact with patients, as it is vital in the diagnosis and treatment of the various forms of anaemia and of leukaemia. Haematologists have the care of patients with these illnesses and also make clinical decisions about their treatment.

Histopathology. Histopathologists examine the structure and abnormalities of macroscopic and microscopic body tissues. The work is mainly of two kinds: first, the examination of tissues from living patients for diagnostic purposes; second, post-mortem examination to determine the cause of death when this has not otherwise been established. Some pathologists can, at times, be called on to carry out post-mortem examinations at the request of a coroner, and a few are regularly involved in forensic work of this kind.

Microbiology. This is the study of disease-producing micro-organisms. The microbiologist examines swabs and other samples of body products in order to isolate and identify the organisms which are causing the trouble. Tests are then carried out on the organisms so that suitable treatment can be recommended. In the light of the test findings, the microbiologist is able to advise, for example, which antibiotics will be effective. The work can also involve investigating outbreaks of infectious disease and identifying the strain of bacteria concerned in order to bring an epidemic under control.

Working Conditions

Most pathologists work in laboratories attached to hospitals but some are employed in other organisations, such as the DSS-financed Public Health Laboratory Service. Laboratory technicians are employed to carry out the many tests that are performed; pathologists advise on the carrying out of the tests and then interpret the results. They also provide the liaison between the laboratory staff and the doctors using their services.

As this is an area where knowledge is increasing fast there is a tremendous volume of new information to be absorbed. The work is obviously most attractive to people who are interested in the scientific aspects of medicine and wish to work in the calmer, nine-to-five world of the laboratory rather than the hurly-burly of night duties and clinical decision taking.

Case Study

A Microbiologist talks about his job

Michael is 31 and employed as an assistant microbiologist (equivalent to senior registrar grade) by the Public Health Laboratory Service.

> I qualified seven years ago and, after 18 months of houseman [house officer] jobs, mainly in general medicine, I decided to go into pathology. I spent the next two years doing a bit of everything before I began to specialise in microbiology. Then I did a year's full-time course at the School of Hygiene and Tropical Medicine in London to get an MSc in medical microbiology. After that I came into my present job. I've taken the first part of my MRC Path and am due to take Part 2 in a few months. If I pass I should, theoretically, be eligible for a consultant post or directorship of a laboratory.
>
> Even as a student I was attracted to the scientific side of things, so I suppose pathology was an obvious choice. The main danger I see is that it's easy to specialise too much, so that eventually you might be working on only one organism. Then the work becomes very enclosed and academic and it's easy to lose a sense of its practical application. I try to avoid too much specialisation by doing small projects on this and that.
>
> The Public Health Laboratory Service is a very kind organisation to work for. It looks after you in the best sort of way and is flexible in allowing you to make career choices. If I pass my Part 2 exam I will probably finish my present job in about a year and then go abroad for a couple of years. At the moment pathology is a shortage specialty, so I should be able to find a consultant post when I return.

Anaesthetics, Radiology and Radiotherapy

These specialties, which do not fit into the broad categories previously described, have certain features in common. They are all concerned with growing technological areas of medical practice, which means that job opportunities are good and research and teaching can play a large part in the work. They are also disciplines in which work patterns, to a large extent, can be predicted in advance and emergencies are few. Part-time posts are therefore possible and this is recognised by the provision of part-time training schemes. Many women doctors have been attracted to these posts because of this. There are more female consultants in these areas of medicine than in any other.

Anaesthetics. Anaesthetists have responsibility for a variety of methods of anaesthesia used for operations, and for pain control in such areas as obstetrics and intensive care. You can choose to work across a wide field acting in conjunction with surgeons and sometimes physicians, or you can specialise in one branch, in which case you are likely to have a more active involvement in the general management of patients.

Radiology. Radiology is concerned with the taking of X-rays. These can be required for diagnostic or investigative purposes and are taken on behalf of many hospital departments. The radiologist, therefore, provides a central information service and will be involved in consultations on a great variety of cases. The work can entail some highly technical procedures as well as the interpretation of X-ray photographs and, sometimes, clinical advice. The radiology department also forms a link between the hospital and local GPs who will often refer their patients there.

Radiotherapy. The radiotherapist works mainly with cancer patients, giving them radiation treatment, and may act as co-ordinator for other forms of treatment as well. Departments are usually based in a few large general hospitals because of the high cost of the equipment used for treatment. There is a high degree of patient involvement, as radiotherapists follow their patients throughout the course of their illnesses, accepting a personal responsibility for them within the context of the whole medical team concerned with the case.

Obstetrics and Gynaecology

Obstetrics is concerned with childbirth and the treatment of women before and after childbirth; it also encompasses family planning and contraception. Gynaecology is concerned with the diseases and hygiene of women. In obstetrics, methods of treatment and attitudes to it have undergone considerable change recently. Technical advances have made detailed monitoring of pregnancy possible but, at the same time, some women have expressed the desire for more personal control over their treatment and a more natural approach. This apparent contradiction has yet to be resolved.

Postgraduate training for obstetrics and gynaecology is well defined. Unfortunately, because of the high incidence of emergency work, there are few part-time posts.

Becoming a Consultant

The competitive and stressful aspects of the time spent in hospital training posts cannot be emphasised too greatly. You will be constantly contending for new posts. Normally, senior house officer posts are held for six months each, across a period of at least 18 months; registrar posts for one two-year period; senior registrar posts for three or more years. After this there is nowhere to go except to a consultancy, as training posts are not usually renewable. Each new post can mean moving to another area and this may cause much disruption, especially if you have a family.

Obviously, there is some wastage during this process, so what happens to those people who opt out? In the past they often went into general practice but now, with new training requirements, this is not so easily done. Community medicine, too, has its own training needs, and not everyone wants to work in community health. It is therefore sensible to decide sooner rather than later if you want to leave the hospital service, so that you feel able to devote the necessary time to alternative training. At present, the greatest wastage probably occurs at registrar level when most people will already have worked for up to two years since registration.

If you reach senior registrar level, the chances are that you will ultimately find a consultant post but, if yours is a popular specialty, you may have little choice where this will be. It is a good idea, both from the point of view of your own training and for your career prospects, to undertake a research project and/or a higher degree. This is often possible at senior registrar level. If you are able to offer this additional experience, you may well increase your chances in the consultancy stakes!

Salary Scales

These are the standard scales from April 1995, the latest available; they are enhanced by additional payments for out-of-hours work and London weighting:

House Officer £13,930–£15,730
Senior House Officer £17,380–£22,060
Registrar £19,705–£29,910
Senior Registrar £22,705–£28,730
Consultant from £40,620.

Finding a Job

Although it is worth making personal inquiries about posts in the specialty or geographical area which interests you, ultimately you will have to wait until a job becomes available. All posts are advertised in the *British Medical Journal*.

Chapter 3

The Doctor in the Community

Introduction

Hospital doctors work in institutions and can, and often do, insulate themselves against the wider implications of their work. A hospital doctor is likely to see a patient for a short time, deal with the problem presented and then proceed to another problem with another patient. It is the problem rather than the individual that is the major concern of the hospital doctor. For doctors who work in the community, however, people are of primary importance. They are involved with individuals' problems, whether personal, social, organisational or environmental. They cannot see illness in isolation and personal contact will be a major factor in their work.

General Practice

More than half of all graduates in medicine enter general practice. The general practitioner has a unique position within the health service. The local doctor's surgery is the only place, except, perhaps, for some accident and emergency departments, where patients present themselves as being, in their own estimation, in need of treatment. General practice is also the most personalised of all the health services, based close to the patients' homes and with opportunities for long-term relationships between doctor and patient. Within this context it is the doctor's job to give early treatment and continuing care for the great variety of problems and disorders presented by patients.

Working Conditions

General practice differs from all other areas of medicine in that it is not salaried. The complicated remuneration system is based on a number of factors. There is a basic allowance for all general practitioners (GPs), capitation payments dependent on the number of patients on a GP's list, and item of service payments. In 1990 a new contract between GPs and the government allowed GPs to derive 60 per cent of their income from target payments, related to cervical cytology uptakes and childhood immunisation take-up rates. More recently group practices which are deemed to be of sufficient size and which have sufficiently advanced administrative methods have the option to become fundholders, which means they have a budget for purchasing specialised services for their patients.

General practitioners have to cope with many moral decisions. Although the underlying principle is that GP services are available for all, individual doctors are not obliged to accept patients on to their lists and can refuse those likely to prove difficult. The social consequences of this are obvious, and though most practices have a policy of accepting everyone in their area who asks to be registered, sadly there are those which do not.

Years ago, the most familiar picture of general practice was of the family doctor working single-handedly from his own home. Things have changed a lot since then, and nowadays approximately 90 per cent of GPs work in group practices. This has many advantages – co-operation over working hours, increased accessibility outside surgery times, the ability to employ more ancillary staff and to offer a more comprehensive service, and the benefits of working alongside colleagues. The group practices are staffed by a 'primary health care team' which includes nurses, health visitors and, often, social workers (care managers). This means that doctors can concentrate on the areas in which their expertise is really needed, knowing that they have all the necessary back-up and that their work will not be done in isolation from the attendant social problems and preventive work.

General practice is challenging because of the variety and unpredictability of the work. With many patients you will have no foreknowledge of their illness and you must constantly be re-focusing on new problems. Most illnesses will be transitory or in their early stages, and you will be faced with the task of diagnosis on very little evidence. The illnesses themselves can cover everything imaginable so you must be able to keep a broad perspective.

Alongside this are the human problems. Patients expect a certain degree of impersonality from hospital doctors, but they look for support and a personal relationship from their GP. However, they often find it difficult to explain the exact nature of their problems, and you must be able to read between the lines when occasion demands. This is obviously the least definable, least teachable aspect of general practice, but it is also very important. Effective birth control provision for teenagers means that there has to be confidence in general practitioners who have to make sure that confidentiality is assured. In this regard, GPs may increasingly see their role changing from that of being providers of a preventive medical service to providers of counselling on patients' sexual lifestyles.

A recent study of complaints against doctors showed that most were not of clinical incompetence but of personal handling – failure in communication.

The great advantage of general practice is its stability. It is rooted in the local community and thrives on continuity. This means that most doctors tend to stay for long periods in the same practice, in contrast to hospital doctors who, at least during the training period, must be constantly on the move. The shorter training period, too, is attractive for people who wish to become settled in their way of life.

Training

Many medical schools have professors of general practice, and students are able to have some first-hand experience of the work during their undergraduate studies. A three-year postgraduate training is statutory for all doctors wishing to become independent general practitioners. This combines hospital posts in relevant specialties with a year's experience as a trainee in general practice. There are two ways of taking this training: either by entering a vocational training scheme, which is a prearranged package of hospital posts and training year, or by a do-it-yourself system of selected posts, which will provide you with relevant experience. Specialties considered suitable for general practice are: accident and emergency, geriatrics, general medicine, paediatrics, obstetrics and gynaecology, and psychiatry. Those who wish to gain experience outside these fields should check with their local training adviser that what they propose is acceptable for accreditation.

During the trainee year, you will work in a practice under the supervision of one doctor who has been selected and briefed for the role. At first you will spend some time sitting in on consultations, but usually you will soon find yourself working alongside the other doctors in the practice. Methods of assessment are still at a formative stage but are increasingly becoming summative. One of the difficulties is that the qualities which make a good GP are not well suited to objective assessment. As things stand at present, the supervising doctor has to testify to the trainee's 'satisfactory completion' of the year but is given few definite criteria on which to make a judgement. It is not necessary to take any examinations, though many people choose to do so. The relevant examination is the Membership of the Royal College of General Practitioners (MRCGP). It attempts to relate to the demands of general practice. It has no practical component and consists of written and oral tests covering all branches of medicine, emphasising such things as problem-solving skills.

In each area there are regional advisers in general practice who will give information and advice about local training schemes. Details of vocational schemes across the whole country can be obtained in a book published by Hawker Publications, 13 Park House, Battersea Park Road, London SW8 4BX. Part-time training is possible in some cases.

Finding a Job

The distribution of GPs throughout the country is controlled centrally in order to try to provide an even spread. There are some areas, notably

London and the South East, which are considered to have their full quota of doctors and it is therefore possible to enter a practice only by filling an already established position. In other places there is a shortage of doctors, and expansion of existing practices or applications to set up new ones will be welcomed.

Jobs are found in two ways. Group practices usually make their own appointments, either by invitation or advertising. Single-handed vacancies are advertised, and the appointments handled by the local Health Service Authorities which have the responsibility for all GP services in the area.

General practice is an area where it is particularly advisable to ensure that your outlook is similar to that of your colleagues. For this reason, whatever the difficulties or pressures of finding a job in an increasingly competitive field, it is necessary to be selective and settle only for a practice into which you feel you will fit.

Jobs are also advertised in the *British Medical Journal*.

Remuneration

A trainee. Trainee GPs earn 15 per cent above the salary of their previous post (April 1993) and receive additional allowances for car and travelling expenses etc.

A principal. In group practices, the distribution of the practice income is a matter which is decided by the partners. New people usually do not get full parity immediately, but should do so in not more than three years.

The average intended net income of a GP was set at £43,165 in April 1995.

Case Study

A General Practitioner considers his trainee year

Mike finished his trainee year a few months ago and now works in a Health Centre.

> When I decided to do medicine I didn't know any doctors. My main ideas came from television and it seemed attractive.
>
> I don't know quite how medical schools select their students. I, in fact, did rather badly in my A levels but I was still offered a place. At my particular medical school we did a survey and found that 86 per cent of the students were from public schools and, of course, there were a lot of doctors' sons. I have no idea why I was accepted!
>
> I wasn't terribly happy at medical school. I found it provided such an isolated form of education and I would have preferred to be at a university. Not a lot of questioning was encouraged. There was just a vast amount of learning, which took away your energy for any form of critical appraisal. I found psychiatry the most interesting subject, and for some time I thought that was what I wanted to do. I then began to see psychiatry as very separate from medicine. In psychiatry, I thought my medicine would not be used so I

began to think about general practice. It is an area where you can develop your own interests, and this appealed to me.

I did my trainee year as a GP after two years in psychiatry, nearly a year on a paediatric ward, and various locums in areas such as old people's medicine and cancer therapy. Locum work is a good way of getting experience. My trainee year was rather a disappointment. I made a bad choice. I had just got married and chose the practice for the convenience of the area rather than for any other reason. I was also not very much in sympathy with my trainer.

Nevertheless, I learnt a lot just by doing the job. I went to the local Postgraduate Centre for a half-day a week and that was good. The course was slanted towards consultations – the doctor/patient relationship – and I found that helpful. For me, this is what matters most about general practice – being involved and getting to know people and their families over a period of time. It is the basis for everything you do, and is helpful in evaluating symptoms. I know that general practice is often thought of as second-rate medicine – you are not a specialist – but the GP does have a specialist contribution to make in terms of assessment of patients' needs and early diagnosis.

It can be quite exhausting emotionally. You come across a lot of cancer patients, people with terminal illnesses; people die and you see bereaved people. And all the time you have the responsibility of recognising illness at an early stage among a heavy work load.

The average consultation time is eight to ten minutes. You can feel quite alone; there is no structure, as in hospitals, to reduce the strain of the personal involvement. Also, being on call can be more of a strain than people realise. The phone might ring at any time, day or night. I go to a Balint group – eight doctors and a group leader – where we discuss difficult cases. Because the doctor/patient relationship is a personal one in general practice, the doctor gets involved too and you have to work out how to keep well yourself and not get worn out by it all. I find the discussions very helpful for this. Being in a health centre also helps. You are much less isolated and have the back-up services of the whole health team. Altogether I'm very biased in favour of general practice. I think it's a good job.

Community Health

The Community Health Service offers services in locally based clinics and much of the work is to do with preventive health care. Although many community health clinics have closed over the last few years because the services they used to provide are more readily available from GPs, there are concerns that vulnerable groups, such as teenage girls requesting contraceptives, may be unwilling to visit their GPs. As recently as 1991, for example, it was found that over 70 per cent of young people under 20 had not consulted their GPs about methods of birth control.

Working Conditions

This is the one area where registered doctors can work without undertaking further postgraduate training, although it may be useful to hold the Certificate of the Joint Committee on Contraception of the Royal Colleges. You will probably be required to work at first under the supervision of a more experienced colleague, and may be required to attend locally arranged short training courses, but such arrangements are informal. In all essentials you will be independent from the outset. Doctors in community health clinics function very much as GPs do, except that they work only in their specialist areas and they cannot prescribe medicines. They can supply contraceptives, which the clinic will stock, but if, while they are examining a patient, they discover any disorders, they must refer the patient back to his or her own GP.

Work in community health clinics is sessional, each session being between two-and-a-half and three hours. Part-time work is therefore easily arranged, and this may be one reason why there is a preponderance of women in the field. Unfortunately, jobs are now being cut during the current 'rationalisation' of services, but there are still some opportunities in this area.

Salaries

The disadvantage of community health is its lack of a career structure. There are just two grades for the community health doctor, with no opportunities for further promotion.

Full-Time Salary Scales (1995)
Clinical Medical Officer £20,775–£28,895
Senior Clinical Medical Officer £29,640–£42,555.

Public Health Medicine

Each district health authority employs public health physicians whose job it is to measure the health needs of the local population, plan appropriate services and evaluate them. Although public health physicians are medically qualified, the work they do is most akin to social administration, and the specialist training they must take reflects this.

Public health medicine, like the hospital service, employs people in training grades, offering permanent contracts only at consultant level. There are about 650 consultants in the field, making this a fairly small working area. There are also district and regional medical officers whose jobs are concerned mainly with management and decision making.

Training

Before beginning specialist training, doctors are required to complete three years of clinical work in a variety of settings, concentrating on relevant aspects of long-term care such as geriatrics and so forth. After this, it is usually possible to be appointed to a two-year registrar post in public health medicine and embark on specialist study. The examination taken by public health physicians is the Membership of the Faculty of Public Health Medicine (MCFM), and, like other postgraduate medical qualifications, it is taken in two parts. Unusually, though, it is taken after a course of formal teaching, the subjects taught being statistics, sociology, epidemiology, economics and management skills. The course is university based and can be taken in two ways: either full time for one year, or as a sandwich course, involving a mixture of both theory and practice. Either way, you will remain in post and be paid your salary throughout. Part 1 of the MFCM is taken by examination and Part 2 is awarded on the basis of a research project.

Working Conditions

Public health physicians do not have direct contact with patients. Their job is to respond to the requests of others – providing information on which decisions can be taken, carrying out research, seeing projects (such as the building of new health centres) through to their conclusion, and liaising with all sectors of the local health service. The public health physician is the main bridge between the doctors and the administrators. You will find yourself attending a lot of meetings, writing reports (which often need the approval of several committees before the recommendations you make can become effective) and generally finding out about the health needs, services and environmental conditions of your area. The amount of freedom you are allowed will vary from one authority to another, but in many places the job can be what you make it, and there will be opportunities to plan and carry out your own research projects.

The field is so wide that most people specialise within it and though everyone is employed in the general role of 'specialist in public health', most will hold responsibility for a particular aspect such as environmental health, social services liaison, information and planning, child health, prevention of disease etc.

If you are interested in the wider implications of medicine, a career in public health medicine is rewarding but you must be prepared to accept the pace at which results are achieved. Mostly this is very slow, as decision-making processes in bureaucratic institutions are extremely lengthy.

Public health physicians sit on district management teams and have a real role to play in the planning of services. There is a strong structure for multi-disciplinary planning teams which can be set up and run by community physicians. These present an opportunity for considering medical problems in a social context and making proposals accordingly. The job is varied and will bring you into contact with a great variety of people, including doctors, working in all sectors of the health service. It may well involve some undergraduate teaching and will have the advantages of a good salary and regular working hours.

Salary Scales and Job Prospects (1995)
Training grades £19,705–£28,730
Consultant in Public Health Medicine from £40,620.

Public health medicine is an expanding specialty, and prospects for employment are, on the whole, good.

Case Study

A Public Health Physician discusses her work

Jenny is the community physician for a socially mixed inner city area which has two teaching hospitals and a well-developed department of public health.

> I did an MSc course at the School of Hygiene in London, because I was interested in social aspects of disease and ways of bringing down the death rate. I also felt critical of the structure of the health service – the fact that it is so doctor-dominated. So I decided to come into public health.
>
> I work as part of the area planning team, which consists of myself, a nurse, a planning administrator, a finance officer and a works officer. There is virtually no contact with patients and often a very long-term feedback of achievements, which I think puts off quite a lot of younger people. On the other hand, the pay is good and you don't have the strain of the immediate responsibilities as you do in clinical work. If you make a mistake, the implications can be serious but you don't see the results of it under your nose!
>
> A lot of the work is research and there are opportunities to follow your own inclinations here. Of course, not all the work goes in the directions you would like.

Chapter 4

Dentistry

Introduction

There are currently 27,472 registered dentists in the UK (January 1995) and over one-third are women. Over 18,000 dentists work in general practice, so dentistry is an attractive career for people who like an independent working situation and the challenge of having total and continuing responsibility for their patients' treatment. Outside general practice, around 1,700 work in the community dental service, 700 in hospitals, and a few are employed by the Forces (see Chapter 5) and large industrial companies.

Training

Training for dentistry is demanding and can be as long as basic medical training. All dentists are now required to undertake postgraduate education to enable them to keep pace with new developments.

As attitudes change, so do the skills demanded of dentists. Much of a dentist's work is highly technical and requires a lot of manual dexterity but today, with the emphasis on preventive work, the dentist is also expected to counsel and educate. People must be persuaded to take proper care of their teeth and be shown how to do this. Anyone thinking of taking up dentistry must feel confident of his or her ability to combine both the technical and the human aspects which will be a part of the work.

There are 14 dental schools run in conjunction with universities in the UK. In addition, certain applicants from the UK are admitted to Trinity College Dublin (to which you should apply direct). All demand similar entrance qualifications – basically, three good A levels in chemistry, physics, maths, biology or zoology or, in Scotland, four Higher Grade SCEs (see Chapter 8). Most schools are, in principle, prepared to accept equal numbers of men and women. Older people who have the Ordinary or Higher National Diploma, but no GCEs, may find that these qualifications are sympathetically considered by most schools, and should write to the Dean or the Admissions Tutor of the individual school to find out if this is so. Application procedures are described in Chapter 8.

Applications to Trinity College Dublin should be made to the Admissions Office.

The full dental course lasts up to six years, but most students are exempted from their first, or pre-dental, year if their A levels are satisfactory. The course proper consists of a pre-clinical year spent studying general and dental anatomy, physiology, biochemistry, histology and, at some dental schools, pharmacology, oral biology, and dental technology and materials science. During the clinical period students work in the laboratory and, under supervision, on preventive dentistry, orthodontics, anaesthetics, oral surgery, periodontology, radiology and community dentistry. A significant part of the clinical period is taken up by general medical studies as a dentist needs a thorough knowledge of the whole body.

There are some opportunities for students, who so wish, to take an extra year studying basic medical sciences, usually between the second and third years of the dental course, to qualify for a BSc degree.

More information, including details of entrance requirements for individual dental schools, can be obtained by writing to the General Dental Council, 37 Wimpole Street, London W1M 8DQ; tel.0171 486 2171.

Registration

In order to qualify as a dental surgeon and to be placed on the Dentists' Register, maintained by the General Dental Council, in accordance with the provisions of the Dentists Act, you must obtain one of the following qualifications:

A first Degree in Dentistry is conferred by a university in the UK or a diploma as a Licentiate in Dental Surgery conferred by one of the Royal Colleges of Surgeons of England and Edinburgh, the Royal College of Physicians and Surgeons of Glasgow. Certain dental qualifications awarded abroad are recognised by the Council as admitting the holders to the UK register without exam. Nationals of an EC country other than the UK who hold an appropriate European diploma are also entitled to registration in the UK. Enquiries should be made to the Council about eligibility of foreign and Commonwealth dentists.

General Practice

Dentists who hold a contract under the NHS may provide a mixture of private and NHS treatment, both across their patient list and within the treatment they provide for one patient. A dentist does not have to accept all patients into NHS care but may choose to see some patients privately and others within the NHS. A patient who is currently registered for NHS care with a General Dental Practice is entitled to receive all the treatment needed under the NHS, but by arrangement with the dentist is entitled to choose to have some (or all) of his or her treatment privately.

Within the NHS, dentists are now paid a capitation fee per registered child patient, which is unrelated to the amount of treatment they provide, plus additional payments for unusual treatments. As far as adults are concerned, part of the fee (that is, payment for continuing care) is paid in a similar way, but a greater proportion of the fee is treatment-dependent.

From their earnings, dentists have to equip and maintain their surgery and pay any staff they employ, for example receptionists or surgery assistants. Being in general practice is therefore rather like running a small business, with all the administrative problems but with all the advantages of independence as well.

There are two points which need to be considered carefully. All newly qualified people will benefit from the support and guidance of more experienced colleagues, and there are many advantages in working in a group practice. Hours can be more flexible, there are more resources available for specialist help, and it is easier to keep pace with new developments when there are opportunities for discussion and the sharing of problems and ideas. In short, a group practice may be better both for the patient and the dentist.

Starting Work in General Practice

Since October 1993, newly qualified dentists have been required to have completed a year's vocational training before they can practise under an NHS contract. Trainees work at the practice of an approved trainer for a salary which starts at around £19,000 (1995). Most young dentists start working as assistants or associates in a group practice. Later, they may become partners and ultimately set up on their own account. There are no set rules for this progression of responsibility. What individuals do will depend on the openings available and their own assessment of what is best for them. Dentists in general practice also have the right to decide what work they will or will not carry out, and must set their own working standards.

Working Conditions

The aim of general practice is to get patients under continuous care – that is, to make them aware of the importance of regular treatment and to make them willing, whatever their fears or reservations, to return for that treatment. This can create a lot of pressure on the dentist, who must constantly be making two kinds of assessment: first, the clinical assessment of the work needing to be done; second, an assessment of the patient and the best manner in which to approach him or her. In any working day this process is gone through many times, usually in the knowledge that a fairly tight time schedule must be kept.

The clinical work undertaken in general practice is wide. There are those who prefer to spend their days doing routine fillings, referring more difficult cases to hospital, but most dentists like the variety and satisfaction of offering a complete range of treatment. If you are going to work in this way, you need to be self-reliant, competent in all aspects of dental care, and able to work under pressure. As many people are apprehensive about dental treatment you must always appear confident and reassuring, however you may be feeling inside, and you will need a good deal of patience and tolerance when dealing with difficult people. You must also be able to work in co-operation with your surgery assistant and any specialist the practice may employ.

Salaries

The incomes of dentists in general practice depend on the demand for their services. With better dental hygiene and higher charges for NHS work, there has recently been more emphasis on preventative work and more complex dental treatments.

The average net income for general dental practitioners is currently (1995) assumed to be about £38,000.

Case Study

A Dental Surgeon gives an account of group practice

Jane works in a large practice in an inner city area. She has been there for three years.

> I trained at Kings in London and qualified five years ago. After qualifying, I spent six months working in a hospital as a house officer. It was a good way to start, because it helped me to build up my confidence within the support structure of the hospital. But in all other ways I much prefer general practice. In hospital, as soon as you see something interesting you have to pass it on to the specialist, and usually you never find out what happens. I think teeth are specialised enough without specialising further within the field. In this practice, we never refer patients elsewhere. We do everything ourselves.
>
> I enjoy the variety of work I get – everything from working with children to doing dentures for old people. I would hate to spend the day doing routine fillings endlessly. There are, of course, the difficult patients – usually the nervous ones who can be quite aggressive. I've often been asked 'Are you sure you know what you're doing? You look a bit young.' Really, people like this are just asking for reassurance, and I look for a way of making them feel they are in control of the situation. I tell them to raise their left hand if anything hurts and that usually works. It *is* very hard work but I get a lot of job satisfaction from it. We are able to set our own working pace and I see about 16 patients a day. That's a fairly low number but I feel that if I went much above that the quality of my work would suffer.
>
> This is a large practice with five full-time and six part-time dentists, including people with special skills. With such a large staff we are able to give a very comprehensive service and to stay open well beyond normal hours. We never turn patients away. We have emergency hours when people can just walk in for treatment, and we find that our patients stay with us, even when they move away from the area. Probably this is because we are one of the few practices in this city to do bridges and crowns on the National Health Service. In fact, we do very little private work – only those things which the Health Service doesn't cover, mainly cosmetic work.

With so many dentists working together, we can have an instant second opinion and a fresh vision on any problems we may have.

Working in a Hospital

Hospital work is salaried, and pay scales (1995) range from £13,930 for house officers to £52,440 for consultants. Conditions of work are also similar, except that there is more emphasis on outpatient clinics and long-stay patients are a rarity.

The DSS recognises four specialties within dentistry – orthodontics, oral surgery, restorative dentistry and, recently, paediatric dentistry – and funds consultant posts in each. Qualified dentists who wish to work in a hospital must follow a similar path to that of hospital doctors, moving through the training grades and combining them with postgraduate study towards their chosen specialisation. Opportunities are, however, limited as the growth rate in hospital dental specialties is virtually nil.

Orthodontics

Orthodontics, at its simplest, is concerned with the straightening of crooked and misplaced teeth. This is done by means of specially made appliances. Undergraduate dental courses cover the basic aspects of orthodontics, and every dentist in general practice should know enough to tackle the simpler work.

There are, however, more complex forms of tooth misplacement which involve far more than a mechanical correction. In these cases specialist knowledge of the development of the jaw is required, and the general practitioner may seek help by referring the patient to a hospital. The hospital staff work closely with local dentists, holding outpatient clinics where the patients referred by them can be seen. Much of the work will be advisory. The problem will be assessed and a report suggesting suitable treatment will be sent to the dentist. Often the work can then be carried out in the general practice surgery, and only the most extreme cases will be treated at the hospital.

Most district hospitals have a consultant orthodontist who has come to the post after eight or so years of postgraduate study. After qualifying, the first step to such a post is a job as a house officer, during which a postgraduate course in orthodontics can be taken. You must then spend a number of years progressing through the training grades, until finally you are eligible for a consultant post. The network of consultant orthodontists is small, however, and you may have to wait longer than the usual time before a post falls vacant.

Orthodontists may also work in general practice, either establishing a surgery with this specialty or dividing their time between several practices in which they give their specialist help. Payment will be on the same basis as for other general practitioners.

Oral Surgery

In oral and maxillofacial surgery the dental and general surgical disciplines meet. It deals not only with the more difficult dental problems but also with accidental injuries to the facial region, facial cancer, abnormalities such as cleft palate, and deformities of the jaw. There are large areas of overlap with other medical specialties, and oral surgeons may work in conjunction with plastic surgeons and ear, nose and throat specialists, among others.

There are about 300 consultant oral surgeons in the UK, many of whom have taken both a dental and a medical training. It is possible to specialise in oral surgery without doing a medical training, but it involves spending longer in the training grades of hospital work and there is today an increasing preference for people with medical qualifications. Those who opt for this specialty have to undergo nine years of basic courses followed by a further eight years or so of postgraduate study and take the Fellowship in Dentistry, a difficult examination with a pass rate of only 10 to 15 per cent.

Case Study

A talk with a Consultant Oral Surgeon

> Most consultants work in district hospitals, dividing their time between one main and two subsidiary hospitals. They probably operate at least three times a week, are on call day and night with a colleague one week out of two, and run outpatient clinics at each of their hospitals. They are, perhaps, assisted by a senior house officer and house officer, and have some responsibility for the further training of their younger staff.
>
> Oral surgery is much the most fascinating and demanding aspect of dentistry. Although it overlaps with general surgery, it demands a practical knowledge of dentistry if the importance of many of the operations is to be understood. We operate on salivary glands, tumours, impacted wisdom teeth, deformed jaws and all kinds of facial injuries. The work is highly specialised and can lead to academic work and research for those people who are interested.

The Community Dental Service

The Community Dental Service was once regarded as the poor relation of the dental profession, but this has begun to change. Many people would like to see its role and importance greatly increased so that it can cater for the dental needs of whole communities. It grew out of the School Dental Service and became the responsibility of the NHS during the reorganisation of 1974. Although its official brief is to treat priority groups, old traditions are slow to die and much of the work has been restricted to treating children and expectant mothers. Recently, treatment of handicapped adults has been added to the categories to be dealt with, but the extent to which this actually happens varies from area to area.

The Service is concerned with public health matters as well as treatment, and fulfils an educational role, running projects, mounting exhibitions and visiting schools, day centres, old people's homes etc. There are also opportunities for research into such things as the effects of fluoridation, the organisation of dental services and so forth. Much of the treatment is carried out in local clinics but there are regular school inspections as well as project-based work which take staff out of the clinics and give a stimulating variety to their working life.

All posts in community dentistry are salaried on scales ranging from £19,705 to £52,440 (1995 figures) so the service represents an attractive alternative for people who do not want to work within the direct payment system of general practice. It would also satisfy those who want to work in a wider community context. Newly qualified dentists can apply for jobs as dental public health officers and, while they are in this post, have the option of taking a postgraduate course in Dental Public Health. The next grade in the career structure is assistant district dental officer, who usually has a specialist area and will also have the opportunity for research, then there is the district dental officer and finally comes the post of consultant in dental public health which carries considerable responsibility for the organisation and general policy of the Service.

Dental Therapists

The Community Dental Service (and, to a lesser extent, hospitals) employ dental therapists who are people who have taken a two-year professional training which qualifies them to treat children under the direction of a dentist. This means that they are not responsible for treatment planning but can carry out simple fillings and extractions and help with instruction about care of the teeth. It is a useful career opportunity for people who lack the academic qualifications for a full dental course but who have a minimum of five GCSEs in English and science subjects and who have a Dental Surgery Assistant qualification. Dental therapists may not work in general practice. At present there is only one training centre – the Dental Auxiliary School, Royal London Hospital Medical College (see p. 68).

Case Study

A Dental Public Health Officer talks about her job

Linda's position is not typical, as her job is a joint appointment between the Community Dental Service and a local teaching hospital. But it does give some interesting indications of the future directions community dentistry may take.

> After qualifying, two-and-a-half years ago, I didn't want to work under the financial pressures of general practice and I definitely wanted a salaried job. I felt that hospital work was too inward-looking, so the community service seemed to answer my needs.
>
> I wanted to work with the elderly and, fortunately, I had this opportunity when a special project was set up to treat handicapped adults. Many elderly

people come into this category. I now have an interesting combination of clinical work, hospital work, home visits and research, which I find very satisfying. At the clinic I treat children and handicapped adults; at the hospital I deal with elderly patients who need dentures; on my home visits I do work for housebound people. I have one day a week set aside for my research. I'm researching the dental needs of elderly people in residential homes and geriatric hospitals, and my findings will be presented for an MPhil or a PhD.

I think that the image of the community service is beginning to change. It used to be thought of as the unpopular branch of dentistry which treated those people no one else was interested in. So it used to get the dregs – people passing through for experience, or dentists who saw it as an easy option. Now, with more back-up from the health authorities and with an expanded role, it is seen as a career. There is bound to be more emphasis on the handicapped in the future, so there will be a lot of new ground to be broken and the opportunities for research and planning are exciting.

Occupational and Industrial Practice

A number of large companies have for many years provided dental treatment facilities for staff at work and a significant proportion of the adult working population is currently served in this way. Although dental services are better known among the larger organisations, there have been instances where groups of smaller companies have joined together locally to share the advantages of a common dental practice. The company usually provides the premises and equipment and pays the dental staff. Treatment is generally provided under the NHS with staff paying the statutory contribution and the fees being assigned by the practitioner to the company.

It is appropriate to stress the importance of the occupational dentist working in close co-operation with the other disciplines in the field of occupational health and not to view the dental service in isolation. A contented and healthy workforce is a productive workforce and the occupational dentist can make a valuable contribution to this.

Career opportunities within occupational dentistry are limited because of the relatively small number of posts available. Posts in occupational and industrial dentistry are advertised in the professional journals; generally a company would expect a successful applicant to have had appropriate experience in general practice, although a broader experience may be an advantage.

Case Study

A Senior Dental Officer discusses occupational dental practice

Bill co-ordinates the dental services which are available to staff working in the head office of a large retail organisation.

I have worked in occupational dentistry for several years, having worked previously in hospital and general practice. In the practice where I work there are approximately 4,500 employees and comprehensive dental care is provided for the benefit of staff. The practice comprises three full-time dentists, one part-time dentist, one full-time oral hygienist, two part-time oral hygienists, five dental nurses, one receptionist, one secretary and one clerical assistant. There are five well-equipped surgeries with a panoramic X-ray machine and an oral hygiene area where patients can be given instruction on a one-to-one basis. Approximately 70 per cent of staff regularly use the facilities provided. There is complete clinical freedom, and the majority of the treatment is carried out under the NHS with staff paying the statutory contribution.

Our dental practice is part of an occupational health department with other health professionals which include doctors, occupational nurses, physiotherapists, chiropodists and an osteopath, and so for me there is the added enjoyment of being part of a team fulfilling a vital role which is valued by the company it serves.

Salary Scales (1995)

General Practice. In general practice you can set your own salary targets, but can expect to earn an average of a little over £38,000.
Community Dentistry. £19,705–£52,440.
Hospital Service. Dentists are paid according to their hospital grade; salaries range from £13,930 for house officers to £52,440 for consultants.

Finding a Job

The main source of job advertisements is the *British Dental Journal*. Apart from this, dental schools occasionally post job advertisements on their notice boards. If you are interested in working in community dentistry it is worth making a direct inquiry to the district dental officer of the area where you would like to work, as there may be unfilled posts not currently being advertised. House officer posts are usually obtained through the member of staff at your dental school who deals with arrangements for postgraduate training.

Chapter 5

Working for the Armed Services and Working Abroad

The Armed Services

The Armed Services offer doctors and dentists either a good financial start and relevant experience for eventual civilian work through a short service commission, or a permanent career with good pay and prospects and a pension at the end of it.

The Armed Services provide self-contained living communities for service personnel and their families and have their own medical facilities. There are opportunities for doctors and dentists, both male and female, to serve either in general practice or in a hospital setting. The scope of the work is similar to that within the NHS, as most of it entails caring for the health needs of servicemen and women and their families. In addition, however, there is the work generated by the activities of the Services themselves – occupational health, aviation medicine, underwater medicine, and exercises in medical practice in war conditions.

Medical and dental officers live in the community into which they are posted, which may be abroad or, in the case of the Navy, on board a ship. All facilities, including housing and recreational and sporting amenities, are provided. You will be an officer of the Service first, wear the appropriate uniform, and be subject to the usual discipline; you will be a doctor or dentist second, but you will be clinically independent and your professional judgement will be trusted. Although there is usually a will to meet your wishes in the matter of postings, this does not always happen and you will, finally, go where you are sent. You will be obliged to serve the length of your commission.

Training

All applicants must receive their undergraduate training in the normal way at a medical or dental school before they begin work with any of the Services. There are financial advantages, however, in deciding to enter one of the Services during your student years by applying for a Ministry of Defence (MOD) cadetship.

Student Cadetships

Each Service operates an identical medical sponsorship scheme (Cadetships) for the last three years before graduation. Acceptance is subject to a successful appearance before a selection board. You are commissioned Second Lieutenant (or equivalent ranks in the RN and RAF), your fees are paid for by the MOD and you will receive a salary which currently (1995) is £9,091 on appointment, rising to £11,368 in your final year. As part of the contract you have to spend a set period after full registration on a six-year Short Service Commission working for the Service concerned. There is little or no commitment to the military during your three-year undergraduate training.

Induction Courses

Each Service has its own short induction course for entrants which covers three main areas: first, general service training, which is an experience of what it is like to be a member of that Service – this includes basic exercises, drill and so on; second, some practice of medical procedures in simulated war conditions; third, a study of your specialist subject as it relates to the activities of the Service.

Postgraduate Training

All the Services have their own hierarchy of medical and dental responsibility, and internal training sessions are arranged for recent entrants. In addition, there are opportunities for postgraduate training which fulfil the requirements of the various Royal Colleges. All Services offer vocational training in general practice and a number of hospital specialties. There is a general emphasis on occupational medicine, and training facilities are good. In most cases, training undertaken during a short commission will be a recommendation for subsequent civilian work.

Rates of Pay

Rates of pay for an officer on a short service commission are comparable with NHS salary scales in junior posts. They range from around £27,534 to £34,089, but it must be remembered that this is a flat rate and there are no extra payments for out-of-hours work. On the other hand, there are various living allowances to compensate for this, including a boarding school allowance for children, in certain circumstances. An additional payment of £1,958 is made to general practice trained doctors. A further £1,076 is made to recognised GP trainers and a further £1,015 to general dental practitioners (1995 figures).

Further information on cadetships, direct entry, conditions of service and remuneration can be obtained by writing to the following addresses:

The Army

Medical
Officer Recruiting
Regimental Headquarters (RHQ) RAMC
Keogh Barracks
Ash Vale
Aldershot
Hampshire GU12 5RQ

Dental
Ministry of Defence, AMD6
Room 42A
Building 21
Keogh Barracks
Ash Vale
Aldershot
Hampshire GU12 5RQ

The Navy

Medical
The Medical Director General (Navy)
Personnel Department
HM Naval Base
Portsmouth
Hampshire PO1 3LR

Dental
Director of Naval Dental Services
Staff of 25th/CNM
Victory Building
HM Naval Base
Portsmouth
Hampshire PO1 3LR

The Air Force

Medical Cadetships
The Director General Medical Services (RAF)
Medical Personnel 1 (RAF)
HQ Personnel & Training Command
RAF Innsworth
Gloucester GL3 1EZ

Medical Direct Entry
Med Personnel 1 (RAF)
HQ Personnel & Training Command
RAF Innsworth
Gloucester GL3 1EZ

Dental Cadetships and Direct Entry
Officer Commanding
Institute of Dental Health and Training
RAF Halton
Aylesbury
Buckinghamshire HP22 5PG

Case Study

A Junior Medical Officer talks about her first RAF posting

Pat was introduced to the crew of the Search and Rescue squadron and to her new role pretty quickly.

> On the most recent trip, I was just about to go down to the married quarters to check on a family when they called me over the storno [radio communication] and said, 'Turn round, come back. They need you.'
>
> At that point they'd been told there was someone who'd had his legs severed in an accident on a ship, so we had to leave extra quickly because he'd be losing vast amounts of blood if this really was the case. I just took my kit in my bag,

jumped in the back of the helicopter and got changed inside.

When we got there, it was the middle of the night and the men were deep down in the hold of the ship. They put the winchman down first and then me. The boat was really throwing around, but we found this pitch-black hole that stank of petrol and diesel, and we got down and found there were two people involved. One was dead, or presumed dead, and the other was injured. I couldn't actually stand up because the boat was throwing itself around so much that I'd just have been thrown against the side of the ship. So I had to kneel down, and even then I was sliding everywhere.

I discovered (working by torchlight) that his leg wasn't severed; it was badly broken, a compound fracture, and someone had put a belt across so he hadn't lost a desperate amount of blood. I gave him some analgesia, strapped him into the stretcher and the winchman started getting him up to the top of the ship.

I did feel pretty ill when I was down there, but you just have to get on with it.

Working Abroad

If you would like to spend some time working abroad, there are opportunities for doctors and, to a lesser extent, dentists, to do much-needed work in developing countries and countries in Eastern Europe. Workers are needed for both short- and long-term commitments, but the average time spent in such posts is around two years.

If travel is your main objective you will probably be disappointed. Many jobs are in remote rural areas, and the demands of the work will leave you with little time to travel far except during your annual leave. The rewards are of a different kind, in terms of the experience you will gain. Your knowledge and training will be a rare commodity and you are likely to find yourself taking on considerable responsibility at a much earlier stage than you would in the UK. Flexibility and resourcefulness will be called for, as you will be working, much of the time, without sophisticated equipment and with an erratic supply of drugs. Many Third World countries are in the process of establishing a health service – often, and probably inappropriately, modelling it on the Western pattern. This can mean that almost the entire health budget is spent on one prestige teaching hospital in the capital city which will be inaccessible to the majority of the population. However, there are interesting projects being set up to provide primary care for rural areas and to explore the most effective ways of improving health. As most illness in developing countries arises from poverty, malnutrition and poor sanitation, education is an important part of medical care. Many projects are community based and doctors will be involved in the training of auxiliary workers who return to their own communities to work. This is challenging work and should be a two-way process, with the doctors learning from the communities they serve what their needs and problems are and how best they can be met.

Finding Work

There are three main kinds of organisation through which work can be found. These are government agencies, volunteer organisations such as Voluntary Service Overseas, and missionary societies. Each offers somewhat different conditions of work and, practical considerations apart, will appeal to people in sympathy with their particular ethos.

Government Agencies

The Overseas Development Administration (ODA) is the part of the Foreign and Commonwealth Office responsible for Britain's overseas aid to developing countries, for global environmental assistance and for assistance to Eastern Europe and the former Soviet Union. The organisation recruits staff for projects funded under British aid. All posts are held on contracts.

In developing countries posts are focused in the following key areas: health sector planning management and financing, population programmes, sexually transmitted diseases, including HIV and AIDS, and communicable disease control. There is a need for health economists, health programme and field managers, health building managers (for hospitals), health planners, health project directors, hospital managers and population experts.

Applicants should have considerable experience in developing countries and, as far as possible, training, management and policy development skills.

Further information can be obtained from the ODA Information Department, Abercrombie House, Eaglesham Road, East Kilbride, Glasgow G75 8EA.

Volunteer Organisations

Voluntary Service Overseas (VSO)

This organisation runs an extensive volunteer programme of which a small part (about 15 per cent) is in the health field.

The projects they sponsor are chosen carefully to fit in with the need for a fairer distribution of services. This means concentrating on local health care which does not rely on expensive technology, and doctors in highly technological specialties are rarely accepted. The emphasis is on a community approach, and a critical attitude towards the organisation of services is encouraged.

Working Conditions

VSO workers are volunteers who are expected to stay for a minimum of two years with their project and are responsible to their immediate employers. They are paid a living allowance at the same rate as their colleagues in the local community and are provided with accommodation. VSO will pay National Insurance, fares, medical cover, insurance, professional fees and small equipment grants. The organisation also contributes to endowment schemes and will post couples where both have relevant skills. Most volunteers live as part of the local community, as their work will be less effective if they are seen as outsiders. This means that knowledge of the local language is vital, and VSO organises preparation courses in England to help with this.

Qualifications Required
Doctors should have at least three years' post-registration experience, preferably in obstetrics, paediatrics, accident and emergency, general medicine, tropical diseases or general practice. Dentists should have two years' post-qualifying experience.

Further information can be obtained by writing to: The Enquiries Unit, VSO, 317 Putney Bridge Road, London SW15 2PN.

International Health Exchange
The organisation provides appropriately trained personnel for programmes in countries in Africa, Asia, the Pacific, Eastern Europe and links health professionals and the organisations working for health improvement in developing countries. It also works to provide greater understanding among health professionals of the health and human resource needs of developing countries and is specifically working to encourage recognition in the UK NHS of the mutual benefits of working in developing countries.

The International Health Exchange runs an international register of health workers as well as short training courses and workshops.

Further details can be obtained from The International Health Exchange, 8-12 Dryden Street, London WC2E 9NA.

Missionary Societies
Missionary societies have been traditionally involved in medical work, and for a long time local mission hospitals provided the only medical care available to large sections of the population in developing countries. Most of the work is still hospital based, usually in quite small units, but there is an increasing tendency towards the establishment of primary health care clinics and the employment of local workers.

Working Conditions
To work for a missionary society you need to be a practising Christian. Missionaries tend to generate a feeling of community and shared faith which can make overseas work a rewarding way of life for believing Christians. Jobs are available on a long- and short-term basis, some in well established settings and some out in the field, developing new services or responding to crises.

Finding a Job
The Medical Missionary Association acts as a clearing house for all posts

available through the UK missionary societies. They publish a magazine, *Saving Health*, which carries a list of health professionals needed overseas in mission settings. Medical Missionary Association staff are available to give individual advice and information about opportunities for work abroad with mission organisations. Each year in May they hold a seminar for medical students planning to spend their 'elective' abroad.

Further information about jobs for doctors overseas with missionary societies can be obtained from the following organisations: The Secretary, Medical Missionary Association, 244 Camden Road, London NW1 9HE; The Christian Service Centre, Holloway Street West, Lower Gornal, Dudley, West Midlands DY3 2DZ; Christians Abroad, 1 Stockwell Green, London SW9 9HB.

Chapter 6

Complementary and Alternative Medicine

Introduction

Complementary and alternative medicine is rapidly becoming accepted as an alternative to conventional medicine and the last ten years have seen a large increase in the number of practitioners in the field. It is no longer regarded as something practised only by a small number of cranks. Most of the disciplines have their foundations in sound principles which, if they were more widely accepted, might ensure better health for the majority of people without recourse to expensive drug treatment. Details of seven very different therapies are given below.

All therapies accept that treatment has to be given holistically, taking an individual's mind and body into account. Consideration of the whole person is regarded as essential to guarantee healing. Illness is seen as a malfunctioning of the body, usually due to some structural imbalance or to an accumulation of harmful substances. This can usually be traced back to an individual's lifestyle, such as unsuitable diet, bad posture, lack of exercise, or build-up of stress. Great emphasis, therefore, is placed on healthy living habits.

Qualities Required of Practitioners

Many doctors who have taken an orthodox medical training decide to train for a particular complementary or alternative therapy; or it is possible to practise after training at a private college without having received orthodox medical training if your standard of education, including science subjects up to A level, is good. You must be completely in sympathy with the philosophy on which the practice is based and for some therapies you must be capable of fairly rigorous study of subjects such as physiology, anatomy, biology, etc. Knowledge of these subjects is necessary as you must be able to make a medical diagnosis of patients in order to determine whether a particular form of therapy is appropriate. Furthermore, you must have the 'feel' and the manual skills for the therapies you wish to practise. You must also have an empathy with people and a real desire to help them.

The Status of Complementary Medicine

Countries vary widely in their official attitude towards complementary and alternative medicine. In the UK hardly any therapies have state recognition. In the USA osteopathy is a mainstream form of medical therapy as it is taught in medical schools, whereas in France it is illegal. In the UK the only therapy currently widely available under the NHS is homoeopathy, although the situation is currently changing. Although there are other therapies such as acupuncture and osteopathy which have to a limited extent recently become available on the NHS, it should be noted that in almost all cases practitioners are operating a private service, charging their patients fees, and students must usually finance their own training.

Organisation of Training and Practice

It can be hard finding one's way around the field. The fact that in most instances there are no controls on either who can set up in practice, or in what constitutes a training for the work, presents difficulties both for would-be practitioners and for patients. To counteract this, the main disciplines have had to set up their own societies or national associations to ensure the preservation of high standards. Only those training schemes which are approved by the main societies are detailed in this book. Students who successfully complete a training course at any one of the colleges listed are accepted as members of the relevant society and are entitled to use its letters of qualification after their names. They are also included in the society's list of qualified practitioners and, in return, must accept the ethical code of practice the society imposes.

It is not advisable to enter complementary medicine by any route other than recommended training establishments. A first imperative is a thorough training and this should be obtained at an approved college. There are dangers inherent in the fact that practice is commercially based, and practitioners should do everything possible to ensure a high standard of professionalism in the service they give.

Natural Therapies

As the body is considered to have the power of self-healing, the job of the therapist is to diagnose and remove obstructions to this self-healing process. This is done through various, very differing, forms of therapy. Many of the therapies in use today derive from ancient medical systems, often from the Far East. Others, of more recent origin (mostly emanating from the USA), make use of high technology to measure the body's responses. Some practitioners use several forms of treatment rather than concentrating on only one, as it is the basic philosophy of holistic healing which is all-important, and inflexibility in attitudes to treatment may be regarded as potentially harmful.

Acupuncture

This is a treatment derived from ancient Chinese medicine, and takes the form of piercing the skin at certain specific points with needles. Conditions which can successfully be treated include migraine, headaches, ulcers and digestive troubles, rheumatic conditions, eczema and other skin ailments, high blood pressure, depression and anxiety states, asthma and bronchitis. Acupuncture can also be used to induce anaesthesia and to treat various forms of addiction. As there is much research into this branch of complementary medicine, acupuncture is being used for an increasing number of diseases.

The therapy is based on the Chinese belief in the dual flows of energy called the Yin and Yang which must be kept in a state of equilibrium in the body. The energy flows along 14 main circuits known as meridians. Equilibrium is maintained by dispelling surplus energy at certain points on the meridian and by shifting energy to deficient areas. Illness is indicative of a loss of equilibrium, and the acupuncturist's job is to restore the balance by piercing the skin at the appropriate points. This involves diagnostic skill and an intimate knowledge of the meridians and the 2,000 or so acupoints at which the skin can be pierced.

Acupuncture can also be used to induce anaesthesia and to treat various forms of addiction.

Practising Acupuncture

Practice arrangements are likely to depend on whether or not you are a registered doctor. Many registered doctors practise acupuncture in addition to their normal medical work and it would appear that opportunities for treating patients under the NHS are beginning to emerge.

If you are a non-registered practitioner, you will most probably have to work in the private sector, alone, in a group practice, or in a health clinic. Through membership of a professional association you can obtain insurance at advantageous rates.

The British Acupuncture Council, Park House, 206–208 Latimer Road, London W10 6RE, acts as a negotiating body for all legal and political matters which affect the practice of acupuncture and it co-ordinates codes of practice, ethical procedures and standards for acupuncture in the UK.

Case Study

An Acupuncturist outlines his career

Richard is a registered doctor who now practises and teaches acupuncture.

Because of family pressures to choose a career with financial security, and my own interest in animals, I decided to become a vet. I did my first two years of pre-clinical studies and it was very interesting. I became very good at table football and learned a bit about veterinary work as well! Then I did an intercalated year for a BSc in neurophysiology, and became very interested in behaviour and pain. After this, the veterinary clinical course was a terrible let-down. It was so turgid, tedious and dogmatic that I decided not to complete it. I decided to switch to medicine. I had to work for a year to get some money together because I had lost some of my grant in the process of changing courses, but this time I carried on to the end.

Sometime while I was a student, acupuncture hit the scene. I remember it well as it was one of the major breakthroughs of my life. There was an article in a Sunday paper about an American in Peking who had anaesthesia through acupuncture for an appendix operation. He was astonished! I thought: 'Here is someone who is objective and he believes in it.' Shortly after this, an acupuncturist visited a patient of mine and talked about his work, and I became more interested. Eventually, I phoned the Acupuncture Association, found out about their course, and combined it with the final year of my medicine course. I qualified in acupuncture in June 1976 and in medicine in the following November.

Then I did my house jobs. One of them was in geriatrics, and one afternoon a week I had an empty outpatients' clinic because all the old people were taken along to a local day centre. So I turned it into an acupuncture clinic instead. All very irregular, but I got my customers – mainly from among the hospital staff.

I had a lucky break. I met an acupuncturist who needed some assistance and later I took over his practice for a year while he was on a sabbatical. He is involved with a radical NHS general practice which operates as a collective and offers acupuncture treatment. I became involved too, and I've worked at the practice for three years now, partly as a doctor and partly as an acupuncturist.

I also do teaching on an acupuncture course. I teach the first medical year and I also teach in the college clinic. This is one of the 'quack' courses, and my association with it makes me unacceptable to the medical acupuncturists. It's all nonsense really. There's not as much difference between the two camps as people normally think. Within orthodox medicine there are so many disciplines and viewpoints, yet they co-exist. In acupuncture it is a parallel situation. The underlying concept is energy – it's a substance. You can consider it from this fundamental view, or be pragmatic. Or you have a third choice. You can be scientific and think one day you will find the nerve patterns to prove it all. In practice, what happens is similar to what happens in orthodox medicine. You try the simple solution first, and if that doesn't work you delve deeper, until eventually you are working with energy patterns, with individuality, and the total person.

Alexander Technique

The Alexander technique is named after Frederick Matthias Alexander, an actor who lived at the beginning of this century and who, as a result of problems with his voice, developed new body postures which he found not only got rid of the problems but also gave him a feeling of well being.

The technique, which is fundamentally a self-help approach, aims to teach people to move freely and to discard the restricted movements and unnatural postures of bodily misuse they have adopted over the years. Practitioners prefer to call themselves teachers of pupils (students are trainee teachers) rather than label themselves as doctors who treat patients. The Alexander technique is primarily used for enhancing physical and psychological good health and well being rather than for directly healing physical and mental problems, but nevertheless has been found to relieve many chronic and even acute conditions such as backache, asthma, hypertension, irritable bowel syndrome and repetitive strain injury.

Teachers usually work on a one-to-one basis with sessions lasting a little under a hour at a time. Training is very comprehensive and lengthy, lasting a minimum of three years.

Healing

Healing has been practised for thousands of years all over the world, as certain people have discovered that they have the power to heal others. It is not a therapeutic system but is based on the belief in a higher reality which orders our physical world, with which we must be in harmony. A break-down of harmony brings about illness. Healers create a bond of empathy between themselves and their patients and allow their energies of mind to flow into their patients and restore them to harmony with the higher reality. They *will* the healing to take place.

Case Study

A Healer talks about her powers

Elizabeth became aware of her healing powers at an early age, and for years sought the path of healing she should follow. Eventually she perfected a preparation of flower potencies which is used world-wide with great success.

> I was a powerful healer by the age of four. At the beginning I practised on animals, and my first notable healing was of a puppy I adored. One night, as I was going to bed, I saw it in terrible distress through poisoning. I ran to it and automatically did what is called 'combing the aura'. By making 'combing' motions around my puppy I saved his life. It is a question of empathy – you feel terribly sorry for the suffering animal or person and this is what brings out your healing ability.
>
> At the age of 17 I started to train as a nurse at St Thomas's. But, very early on, I discovered vivisection and I was so horrified that eventually I couldn't finish the course. That made me turn my back on conventional medicine. Instead, I studied alternative therapies – some in considerable depth. None matched up to what I was looking for. When I was 44 I got direct clear intelligence which, over the course of years, led me to the method by which the energies given off by flowers can be radically modified and stored in simple preparations – which then act as batteries containing the energy.

> My preparations are unique. Drugs work on the physical body and homoeopathic medicines on the psychic body (that is, on radiations or emanations from the physical body). My flower potencies do neither. What they do is to remove the psychological and emotional blocks stopping a being from accepting the gifts that God continually gives. A by-product of these gifts is health.
>
> The energy in the preparations cannot be analysed chemically but can be measured on a voltmeter and it is the energy which is the active principle that does the healing. Because the preparations have no bad side-effects they are a simple, safe, self-therapy. They can remove any infective or diseased condition and have proved effective in cases of the most severe injury, and of terminal cancer. They ease and smooth the path of the dying. I have never known them to fail if correctly used.

Herbal Medicine

Herbal medicine as practised today is the accumulation of many centuries of wisdom. Many plants are used – in some instances the flowers, stems and roots – as well as parts of trees and seaweed. They are used both to heal and to ensure continued good health. Trained medical herbalists prescribe plant-based remedies in the form of lotions, ointments, poultices, syrups, essential oils and tablets. In the case of illness, these are intended to restore the body's equilibrium and help it to heal itself. Medical herbalists question their patients at length about their medical and family histories, allergies, reactions to drugs, diet and general lifestyles. They will then prescribe medicines according to individual needs and not solely on the basis of specific illnesses. The medicinal herbs may be for eliminating unwanted substances from the body, for detoxification or for promoting good health in an already healthy body.

Homoeopathy

Homoeopathy is practised either by a number of medical doctors who have undertaken specialist training in homoeopathy and who may be working for the NHS, or professional homoeopaths who are qualified in this specialty only. The former may use a combination of homoeopathic and mainstream medical remedies, while the latter will use only homoeopathic remedies. Homoeopathy is a treatment of the whole person, and symptoms are seen as 'expressions of disharmony within the whole person'. When homoeopathic doctors and homoeopaths take a case history they pay attention not only to the patient's description of the symptoms but also to his or her personality, likes and dislikes. Because they realise that individuals react to illness in different ways, they will not always give the same treatment for the same illness. Disease is treated by the use of very small amounts of a substance, a minimal dose, that, in healthy persons, produces symptoms similar to those of the condition being treated. Remedies are produced from plant, mineral and animal sources and may be in the form of pills, powders, granules or tinctures and, because they are administered in minute doses, they produce no side effects. The healing process is gentle and designed to activate the body's own restorative powers.

Hypnotherapy

Hypnotherapy uses hypnosis to tap into the unconscious to achieve behavioural change. Hypnosis is a state of altered consciousness during which the unconscious mind becomes receptive to suggestion. Hypnotherapy has had many successes in the treatment of physical conditions where there is probably a strong psychological element. Examples are psychosomatic illnesses such as hysterical paralysis or kleptomania, or conditions caused by stress such as migraines, nail-biting, bed-wetting, eating disorders and skin problems. The therapy is also recommended for treating problems in the gastro-intestinal tract, such as colitis, which are thought to be stress-related. It has also proved effective in treating insomnia and anxiety as well as phobias, such as fear of spiders, exams, heights or flying, and addictions and dependency states, such as alcoholism, smoking and gambling. In dentistry, the technique is used for analgesia.

Most hypnotherapists work either on their own or in private practice, but there is increasing scope for working in hospitals.

Osteopathy

Osteopathy is a system of manipulating the bones and tissues to relieve pain and tension. The osteopath corrects dysfunctional movements in the body and allows the natural healing to take place. Many people think of osteopaths as people who may cure their backache when all else has failed, but osteopathy can have more far-reaching results. Although a lot of the treatment is concerned with manipulation of the spine, it can extend to the whole of the body and give benefit in cases of apparently unrelated illness. Recent research suggests that muscular and skeletal disorders can create abnormal strains on nerves and blood vessels which, in turn, can have an effect on such functions as digestion, respiration and circulation. So, although the primary function of osteopaths is to relieve pain, they may also be able to alleviate a wider range of disorders.

The Osteopathy Act 1993 ensures the validity of a regulatory body which will stop unqualified practitioners practising in the field.

Working as an Osteopath

If you decide to practise this form of therapy, you will use a complex system of manipulation for which you will need a sound knowledge of anatomy. Before you decide on a course of treatment, however, you will take a full case history of your patient, much as a doctor does, and make a full clinical examination of the patient's present condition. You will note the configuration of the spine and test the patient's ability to walk and move his or her limbs. Only when you have all the necessary evidence and are able to decide that manipulation will work, will you begin the appropriate course of treatment. Although manipulation can be helpful in many cases, there are disorders for which it would be disastrous, for instance if the prognosis is osteoporosis (brittle bones) or if the joints are inflamed. For this reason, basic clinical knowledge is needed for diagnostic purposes and, if you are in any doubt yourself, you must refer your patient to someone who can provide the necessary back-up.

Case Study

John has been teaching yoga for many years and is now taking a part-time course in osteopathy.

> During my years of yoga teaching I have been working out ways of opening up the body and freeing energy. What I do is to stretch people out and achieve a very deep, very powerful stretching of the muscles. When I am qualified as an osteopath I will combine this with osteopathic techniques. It is interesting work – everything comes into it, including psychology. You can't divorce bones from the brain. The idea is seeing someone as a total person. I believe that the body has its own healing force and for this reason I see education as my primary function. I teach exercises first and do manipulation second. Only in cases of extreme pain is manipulation the priority.
>
> A lot of people become ill because they have no safety valves. My job is to teach people how to relax deeply – both physically and mentally. Most people don't even know how to breathe. PE in schools would be an opportunity for this kind of education, but in fact no one teaches you about your body and how to keep it functioning....
>
> Most patients who come to osteopaths do not need much medical diagnosis but there are always the exceptions. As well as the osteopathic, or structural, diagnosis the osteopath is qualified to make a medical diagnosis, but obviously doctors are better at it because they are doing it all the time. There ought to be much more contact between the two sectors, much more working together. That would be the best hope for the future.

For further information about complementary or alternative medicine and the different therapies available, as well as education and training and information about registering organisations, please refer to *Working in Complementary and Alternative Medicine* by Loulou Brown, published by Kogan Page, or contact the Council for Complementary and Alternative Medicine or the Institute for Complementary Medicine (addresses on p 95).

Chapter 7

Mental Health

Introduction

The field of mental health is wide and difficult to define. Problems may range from temporary emotional difficulties to physiological learning difficulties. In general the area is characterised by being very labour-intensive and staffed by people who have trained in a variety of disciplines. Treatment is provided in a number of different settings funded by several agencies.

Treatment of mental health difficulties have traditionally followed particular theoretical models. The key models, which differ widely in their approach to particular problems, are the following:

(a) the medical model which views mental disorders as *illnesses* which can be physiologically tested;
(b) the cognitive model which sees disorders as arising through *negative thought patterns*. Treatment centres on challenging negative thoughts;
(c) the behavioural model which does not speculate on mental processes at all; rather, it selects only observable *behaviour* as the problem. Treatment centres on reinforcing appropriate behaviours;
(d) the social model which investigates underlying *social causes* (for example, divorce, poor housing). Treatment requires changes in living conditions;
(e) the psychodynamic model which views repressed *unconscious conflicts* as the source of the disorder. Treatment involves making these hidden conflicts conscious.

To a large extent the mental health professions follow on from these theoretical models, although in recent years there has been a move by all who operate in the field towards integration and the development of eclectic methods to obtain the best treatment most relevant for a particular client.

While the work you do will be dictated to an extent by the setting, it will vary according to your training and personal inclinations.

Work Settings

As with other forms of health provision, treatment is given in two main settings: in hospitals and in the community. Following the Mental Health Act 1983, the overwhelming trend is a move to work in the community with a closure of long-term mental hospitals. This applies to all forms of care, from emotional problems to people with learning difficulties. Services are provided by the Health, Education and Social Services, a variety of voluntary associations, and the private sector. Each tends to employ people who have trained within a particular discipline, though this is not an absolute rule. In 1991 the Care Programme Approach was introduced, providing individual care plans for people using the specialist mental health services, while in 1993 Care Management was introduced into the social services which involved the appointment of care managers (social workers) to assess individuals' needs

Training and Professional Functions

The main functions practised within mental health are assessment, counselling and various forms of psychotherapy, and drug and ECT treatment. People come to the work through the following routes:

Psychiatrists are medically qualified people who choose to specialise in psychiatry. They follow the postgraduate training pattern described in Chapter 2 and take the membership examination of the Royal College of Psychiatrists (MRC Psych). In accordance with the Mental Health Act, many psychiatrists now work in community teams. Psychiatrists are the only practitioners eligible to prescribe medication. It is quite common for psychiatrists to take a further training in psychoanalysis (see p 89) at a later stage in their career.

Psychotherapists work in situations where treatment is given through some kind of talking, whether one-to-one, with family units, or in groups. They concern themselves with understanding the problems within the individual's psyche, or a family's relationships, or with group dynamics. A common training for psychotherapy is a degree in Humanities, followed by a professional training. This always entails a course of personal insight training or analysis and many people come to the work because of their own experience of such therapy. Doctors wishing to become psychotherapists will receive postgraduate training (and advice on it) through the training structure described in Chapter 2.

Recent developments in psychotherapy include brief, time-limited psychotherapies available within the NHS. Cognitive Analytic Therapy (CAT), for example, is an integrative therapy which uses an eclectic mix of cognitive, psychoanalytic and behavioural strategies to enable clients to develop specific tools with which a person can understand and change maladaptive coping patterns. CAT has been used in many NHS settings, ranging from general mental health to specialist, forensic and eating disorders. Currently, CAT training is rapidly expanding throughout the UK. Another psychotherapy, Psychosynthesis, works towards integrating different therapeutic methods, with a particular emphasis on the concept of 'The Will'.

Psychologists are graduates in psychology who have taken further professional training to become either clinical or educational psychologists. Work experience is necessary before embarking on any professional training; for educational psychologists this must be in teaching while for clinical psychologists work experience requires clinical psychiatric experience. Psychologists have, until recently, been concerned mainly with assessment and testing and have therefore worked largely in an advisory capacity with those people actually giving treatment. Historically there has been a tendency for psychologists to work with people who have emotional problems, using behavioural and cognitive techniques. Psychologists can be employed in a variety of settings, but are usually taken on by the Health or Education Authorities.

Unlike other practitioners in the mental health field, psychologists are equipped to develop new treatment strategies. Behavioural operant conditioning methods for people with learning difficulties are a recent development that has proved highly successful for reducing problem behaviours.

Psychiatric social workers are people with social work qualifications who can choose to specialise in mental health by taking additional professional training. Such people often work in community settings where their background enables them to work with whole families. Unlike other workers in the health care professions, social workers have important legal powers and responsibilities. These particularly concern work with children where, for example, social workers may be required to take out care orders to restrict parent access.

Counsellors are often employed in educational establishments, giving advice and back-up to students with personal problems and working mainly on the level of interpersonal relationships. Many are trained teachers who may have taken one of the counselling courses available. Counsellors are employed under various guises. Some are called counsellors, some are known as young people's advisers, and others fulfil this function within the wider brief of the post of education welfare officer.

Outside education, job opportunities are limited in the present economic climate, though there is a demand for part-time voluntary counsellors to work with community groups dealing with a wide range of problems.

Working in Hospitals

Hospitals divide into two main groups: those dealing with learning difficulties and mental illness, whether chronic or acute, and general hospitals which have departments of psychiatry often handling less severe cases, mainly in the outpatient clinic. The work encountered in the two groups will be very different and the nature of the work will depend both on the problems presented by individual patients and on the perceptions and aims of the staff dealing with them. Long-term in-patient work has been radically changed by the effects of the Mental Health Act 1983 and the multi-disciplinary team approach whereby particular therapeutic roles and responsibilities (such as drugs, psychotherapy, behavioural work) are allocated to particular members of the team.

Case Studies

A Child and Family Psychiatrist reviews her work

Ruth combined her training with raising a young family, and now, 13 years after she qualified, is looking for a part-time consultancy.

> I went into medicine because I had an interest in people's emotions and ideas about treating the whole person. As a student I was very involved in psychiatry during two out of three of my clinical years. We had a well-known psychoanalyst teaching at the time and he had a great personal influence on me. He was very uncompromising in his approach and insisted that we gain a helpful understanding of *all* aspects of the patient's life. We also did some individual psychotherapy under supervision.
>
> When I qualified, initially I was intending to go into general medicine as a route to psychiatry, but the next thing that happened was that I became pregnant *and* did a job in paediatrics all at the same time.... I decided to combine my two interests and go into child psychiatry but the great question was: how? That was 12 years ago, and at that time the training structure was only thinly mapped out. As hospital posts were virtually an impossibility for me I felt at a standstill and didn't know how to pursue what I knew I ultimately wanted to do. I took up the opportunity of doing some sessions in paediatrics, which were quite useful on the developmental side, and then, two years later, had my second child. After that I spent two years working on a research project on developmental paediatrics and emotional problems, got the project published, and became a school doctor. By this time, it was obvious to me that the pathway to child psychology was via adult psychiatry, which is concerned mainly with mental illness rather than with people with problems. My third child was born around this time and I got myself a part-time registrar post in a mental hospital. With a gap for maternity leave, I carried on with this part-time training both in the mental hospital and in a district general hospital for three years. During this time I took my MRC Psych and then was appointed to a part-time senior registrar post in child psychiatry, in which I have been for the past four years.
>
> My main interest now is in family therapy. There's a lot of unexploited scope to help people with problems mainly through talking and looking at the family and social environment. Most children are referred because of disturbing emotional states such as unhappiness or anxiety, for behaviour problems like stealing, disobedience or truancy, or because they present bodily symptoms – soiling, abdominal pains, eczema and asthma, and so forth. It is very common to express emotional difficulties in these ways. As I see it, there's usually no point in treating the symptoms – you have to go back to what got them there. That's why I like working with the whole family, because they are all likely to be involved.

A talk with a Consultant Child Psychiatrist

I work in a rural area, and am one of three consultant child psychiatrists in the county. There are nine consultants in adult psychiatry and, although our work areas do not usually overlap, we all co-operate over on-call duties. Otherwise, my time is divided between a residential child psychiatric unit, a hospital for the mentally subnormal, two sessions working in social services assessment centres, and the remainder in outpatient clinics of local hospitals.

It is a working life with a lot of variety, and I think this is one of the attractive aspects of psychiatry. I am working not only in different settings but with people as individuals, and no two people are alike. So the work is non-repetitive. I also work with multidisciplinary teams and we each bring our own expertise to bear on the problems our patients present.

My main involvement is with the child psychiatric unit. We take between 24 and 40 children from the age of five until 19, and aim to provide them with an environment for living in which their problems can be treated. All have fairly extreme forms of psychosis or neurosis. We have family accommodation, at present occupied by a mother and her six-year-old son, which enables us to treat a family as a unit when other forms of treatment have failed or simply to offer accommodation to parents should they wish it. We also have a school which the children attend, and a team of workers consisting of myself, nursing staff, social workers, therapists and teachers. We discuss each child every six weeks with the parents present, and together we decide how treatment should proceed. We don't work according to set theories. We are open-minded and will try anything which we think will prove effective.

The mental subnormality hospital has a preponderance of adults. There is an increasing tendency for handicapped children to be cared for in the community, which means that those remaining in the hospital are mainly very severely handicapped. The hospital is divided into two units, and I have responsibility for one of them, both adults and children. My role is one of general medical and psychiatric supervision of the team of workers, in the sense of both general and individual management of patients, their treatment, and training programmes.

Working in the Community

The main forms of mental health care in the community are provided by the Health, Education and Social Services, MIND, a variety of voluntary bodies (notably Arbours and Relate), and by private clinics. Recently, there has been a sharp increase in growth in provision of services in the community. The move to the community was intended to provide less stigmatised and more integrated facilities than the old 'asylums' could provide. In some instances, however, shortages of funds have resulted in diminished standards of care. The work takes place in child guidance clinics, health centres, family welfare clinics, educational establishments, some general practices, and clinics run privately or by voluntary bodies. In the case of people employed by health authorities, there are many areas of overlap between hospital- and community-based work. Psychiatrists and psychologists, for instance, may be attached to a hospital but do much of their work in a community setting. The methods of treatment are similar to in-patient work, although it is hoped that the stigma and isolation of the hospital will be avoided. But the lack of availability of provision of treatment (such as drugs and counselling) owing to depleted funds has been a key issue of concern.

Case Studies

A Psychotherapist discusses her work

Pam works for a voluntary group providing various forms of psychotherapy for women within a feminist framework.

> Our group started life in a basement through the initiative of two feminists who saw a need for a provision specifically for women. They advertised in the feminist journals and the response was overwhelming.
>
> Now, five-and-a-half years later, we have five therapists and are in new premises with six rooms – two for group work and four for individual therapy. We are financed mainly by fees, which we charge on a sliding scale, but we do have some funding from Partnerships and various charitable trusts which enables us to widen the scope of our work and undertake projects which are broadly 'educational'.
>
> Our work is mainly of five types. We offer long- and short-term therapy, organise workshops, start and support self-help groups and run training courses for people already working in the field. We find the greatest demand is for individual therapy, either to help women with ongoing problems or to assist in the short term with people experiencing crises. Workshops are usually theme-related, under headings such as 'Women and Anger', 'Mothers and Children', or 'Sexuality', and in self-help groups we have done a lot of work on compulsive eating. We also help mixed groups of women who want a structure for getting together and sorting out their problems. We see our training courses as a topping-up for people who are already trained. Our view is that to train as a therapist you must train broadly, and we, after all, are specialists.
>
> Nowadays there is a choice of professional training courses run by places like the Tavistock Clinic and Arbours, but when I trained over 15 years ago, these weren't in existence. I took a Mental Health course at the LSE. This entailed doing therapy under supervision and having personal analysis. Until I came here I worked in NHS clinics as a psychotherapist, and much of my work here has been in psychotherapy. At the moment I am developing my interest in counselling, which is concerned with interpersonal relationships as opposed to problems within the psyche. I am planning a course on 'Counselling by Women for Women' – obviously a woman-to-woman counselling relationship is very different from a man-to-woman one, and I want to explore this through the course.
>
> We have expanded over the five-and-a-half years of our existence, but still cannot cope with the demand. There are places where adults seeking individual therapy can go, both under the NHS and privately, but finding them can be rather like looking for a needle in a haystack.

An Education Welfare Officer reviews her job

Sue is a school-attached worker and deals with secondary school age pupils who have no school counsellor. She therefore provides this service.

> I operate in two distinct ways: as a worker with families who are usually referred to me for truancy problems, and as a counsellor for children with

personal problems. I took this job after completing teacher training so I have learnt my counselling techniques on the job. The Authority runs an induction course but I didn't find it very useful.

Some children are referred to me by the teaching staff, but often children come to me of their own accord because I am in a neutral position and they can expect confidentiality. This is very important. They do not want their teachers to know about the things they tell me. I get all sorts of problems thrown at me. A child will burst in, saying, 'Please help me, I never want to go home again'. Some are quite disturbed – temporarily. Most problems boil down to conflicts with parents or difficulties in sexual relationships. I never take a moralistic standpoint, although if I am asked straight out what I think, I will give an opinion.

I prefer to spend the first few sessions getting children to talk out the problem, offering some suggestions for ways of thinking about it so that perhaps they will analyse it and find solutions themselves. Very often these problems have commonsense answers. Occasionally I will set specific tasks, especially in cases involving conflicts which arise for particular reasons. I will, for instance, ask a child who is clashing with parents because of untidiness to be especially tidy for one week and see how that changes the situation. I will also give advice if this seems appropriate.

The patterns of self-referral are interesting. Girls will come alone to see me; boys come in groups, full of bravado, and will very rarely admit to problems. They have obviously come for a reason, but it is very difficult to break through and identify it.

A large part of this job is recognising problems. You have to be able to make a quick assessment – is it a personal, educational, or social problem or do the problems, in fact, overlap? You have to be able to judge when you can help and when you should refer to another agency. We need to know a little about a lot!

Salary Scales

Pay generally relates more to the training and discipline rather than to the mode or style of work you are doing. The disciplines of psychiatry, psychology and social work have their own career and pay structures on a national basis. Counselling, psychotherapy and psychoanalysis have pay structures more determined by fund-holder offers or private personalised charge rates.

Finding a Job

Most job advertisements appear in the journals of the various professional associations. It is also advisable to look at Wednesday's *Guardian* and on hospital billboards. The best way to find a job might be through networking with professional colleagues.

Chapter 8

Professional Qualifications and Training Courses

Medical and Dental Undergraduate Courses

All these courses are run in conjunction with universities, and applications are made through the Universities and Colleges Admissions Service (address on p. 92). You should consult *The UCAS Handbook* for the relevant year of entry: this will provide details of the admissions procedure and how to apply. Applications are normally made between 1 September and 15 December of the year preceding the year of entry. Prospective students are strongly advised to obtain prospectuses of the universities, schools and colleges in which they are interested before making their application, as courses and entrance requirements vary.

Entrance Requirements for Medical and Dental Courses

Entrance requirements are of two kinds: the general requirement to enter any degree course of an institution of higher education and those required for the course of your choice. Full details (subjects, grades, examining bodies etc) can be found in *University and College Entrance: Official Guide*, available for consultation in most libraries, or details of an individual institution's requirements will be set out in its prospectus.

All institutions accept for general requirement the A-level subjects developed by the Nuffield Foundation Science Teaching Project. They also accept biology, chemistry and physics in individual course requirements. Physical science may be an acceptable alternative to physics and/or chemistry.

Many universities require a GCSE (or equivalent) pass in English language.

If you are applying for a place at an Oxford or Cambridge college, please note that you cannot apply to both universities in the same admissions year. The admissions system for medical students has recently changed for these two universities. If you are applying to Oxford, submit a complete Oxford Application Card to the Oxford Colleges Admissions Office by 15 October. If you are applying to Cambridge, submit a completed Preliminary Application Form to the Admissions Tutor of the Cambridge college listed as your first choice, or, in the case of an open application, to the Cambridge Intercollegiate Applications Office by 15 October. If, however, you are already a graduate you can bypass UCAS and apply direct to the particular college of your choice.

Some institutions will waive entrance requirements in the case of mature students. University policies on this matter are outlined in *University and College Entrance* and you should make enquiries of individual institutions. The usual A level requirements and length of study are given after the addresses.

Pre-medical and Pre-dental Courses (1st MB, 1st BDS)

There are some opportunities for students who have taken unacceptable combinations of subjects at A level (or equivalent) to qualify for entry to a full medical or dental course by taking a first MB course in science subjects. Entry requirements are similar to those for university courses generally, but some evidence of the study of sciences, either at GCSE or A level, is usually required. Universities offering these courses are marked in the list with an asterisk.

Medical Schools

Aberdeen: University of Aberdeen, Admissions, Faculty of Medicine, Regent Walk, Aberdeen AB9 1FX; ABB; 5FT.

*Abertay, Dundee: Admissions Officer, Faculty of Medicine & Dentistry, Dundee DD1 4HN; ABB; 5/6FT.

Belfast: Queen's University of Belfast, The Dean, The Medical Faculty, University Road, Belfast BT7 1NN; AAB; 5FT.

Birmingham: University of Birmingham, Assistant Registrar, The Medical School, Birmingham B15 2TJ; ABB; 5FT.

**Bristol*: The Registrar and Secretary, Senate House, Tyndall Avenue, Bristol BS8 1TH; ABB; 5/6FT.

Cambridge: University of Cambridge, The Clinical School Offices, School of Clinical Medicine, Addenbrooke's Hospital, Hills Road, Cambridge CB2 2QQ. (Enquiries about admission to the course of pre-clinical study should be directed to: Cambridge Intercollegiate Applications Office, Kellet Lodge, Tennis Court Road, Cambridge CB2 1QJ); AAA; 5/6FT.

Edinburgh: University of Edinburgh, Associate Dean (admissions), Medical School, Edinburgh EH8 9AG; AAB; 5/6FT.

Glasgow: University of Glasgow, The Convenor, Admissions Committee, Faculty of Medicine, Glasgow G12 8QQ; ABB; 5FT.

Leeds: University of Leeds, Admissions Officer, Faculty of Medicine, Leeds LS2 9JT; ABB; 5FT.

Leicester: University of Leicester, Senior Tutor for Admissions, Medical School, Medical Sciences Building, University Road, Leicester LE1 7RH; ABB; 5FT.

Liverpool: University of Liverpool, Admissions Secretary, First Floor, Duncan Building, Royal Liverpool Hospital, Prescot Street, Liverpool L7 8XW; ABB; 5FT.

London: Charing Cross and Westminster Medical School, The Secretary, The Reynolds Building, St Dunstan's Road, London W6 8RP; 21-22 pts; 5FT.
King's College School of Medicine and Dentistry, The Secretary, Bessemer Road, London SE5 9PJ; BBB; 5/6FT.
Queen Mary and Westfield College, Admissions Office, Mile End Road, London E1 4NS; BBB; 5FT.
Royal Free Hospital School of Medicine, The Registrar, Rowland Hill Street, London NW3 2PF; BBB; 5/6FT.
St George's Hospital Medical School, Admissions Officer, Cranmer Terrace, London SW17 0RE; ABB; 5FT.
St Mary's Hospital Medical School (Imperial College), The Secretary, Norfolk Place, London W2 1PG; BBB; 5FT.
United Medical & Dental Schools of Guy's & St Thomas's Hospitals, Admissions Officer, UMDS – St Thomas's Campus, Lambeth Palace Road, London SE1 7EH; BBB; 5FT.
University College London Medical School, The Tutor to Medical Students, Faculty of Medical Sciences, Gower Street, London WC1E 6BT; BBB; 5FT.

(Note that each London medical school counts as a separate choice on the UCAS application form.)

Manchester: University of Manchester, Tutor for Admissions, Medical School, Stopford Building, Oxford Road, Manchester M13 9PT; ABB; 5/6FT.

**Newcastle*: University of Newcastle upon Tyne, Administrative Assistant (Admissions), The Medical School, Framlington Place, Newcastle upon Tyne NE2 4HH; ABB; 5/6FT.

Nottingham: University of Nottingham, Admissions Officer, Medical School, Queen's Medical Centre, Nottingham NG7 2UH; ABB; 5FT.

Oxford: University of Oxford, The Senior Assistant Registrar, Oxford University Medical School, John Radcliffe Hospital, Headington, Oxford OX3 9DU; AAA; 6FT.

St Andrews: Admissions Officer (Medical Science) Faculty of Science, College Gate, St Andrews KY16 9AJ; ABB; 3/4FT.

Sheffield: University of Sheffield, The Sub-Dean for Medical Admissions, Medical School, Beech Hill Road, Sheffield S10 2RX; ABB; 5FT.

Southampton: Senior Registrar, Faculty of Medicine, Southampton SO9 5NH; ABB; 5FT.

**Wales*: University of Wales, College of Medicine, The Registrar and Secretary, Heath Park, Cardiff CF4 4XN; ABB; 5/6FT.

Primary Qualifications awarded by Royal Colleges and by the Society of Apothecaries in London

Licence of the Royal College of Physicians of London, The Diploma of Membership of the Royal College of Surgeons of England. Examining Board in England c/o Royal College of Surgeons of England, Lincoln's Inn Fields, London WC2A 3PN. The Licence and Diploma are not granted separately.

Diplomas of the Royal College of Physicians of Edinburgh, The Royal College of Surgeons of Edinburgh, the Royal College of Physicians and Surgeons of Glasgow and the Society of Apothecaries of London. The examinations for the Triple Qualification of the Scottish Colleges are conducted by the Committee of Management, Nicholson Street, Edinburgh EH8 9DW and 242 St Vincent Street, Glasgow G2 5RJ.

Details of these awards are given in *British Qualifications* (Kogan Page) or may be obtained from the administering bodies.

Dental Schools

(Pre-dental schools are marked with an asterisk. The usual A level requirements and length of study are given after the addresses.)

**Abertay, Dundee*: Admissions Officer, Faculty of Medicine and Dentistry, Dundee DD1 4HN; BCC; 5/6FT.

Belfast: Faculty of Medicine, Queen's University Belfast, University Road, Belfast BT7 1NN; ABB; 5FT.

Birmingham: Dental School, Birmingham University, St Chad's Queensway, Birmingham B4 6NN; BCC; 5FT.

**Bristol*: Dental School, Bristol University, Bristol BS1 2LT; BBB; 5/6FT.

Glasgow: Undergraduate Admissions Office, Glasgow Dental Hospital, 378 Sauchiehall Street, Glasgow G2 3JZ; BBB; 5FT.

Leeds: School of Dentistry, The University of Leeds, Clarendon Way, Leeds LS2 9LU; BCC; 5FT.

Liverpool: School of Dental Surgery, The University, Pembroke Place, PO Box 147, Liverpool L69 3BX; ABB; 5/6FT.

London: Guy's and St Thomas's, United Medical and Dental Schools, Guy's Hospital Medical School, London Bridge SE1 9RT; BBC; 5FT.
*King's College School of Medicine and Dentistry, Denmark Hill, London SE5 8RX; BCC; 5FT.
Queen Mary and Westfield College, Mile End Road, London E1 4NS; BBB; 5FT.

(Each London dental school counts as a separate choice on the UCAS application form.)

**Manchester*: Turner Dental School, Higher Cambridge Street, Manchester M15 6FH; BBB; 5/6FT.

**Newcastle*: Dental School, Framlington Place, Newcastle upon Tyne NE2 4BW; BCC; 5/6FT.

**Sheffield*: School of Clinical Dentistry, Charles Clifford Dental Hospital, Wellesley Road, Sheffield S10 2SZ; BCC; 5/6FT.

**Wales*: Dental School, University of Wales, College of Medicine, Heath Park, Cardiff CF4 4XY; BBC; 5/6FT.

Other Registrable Qualifications

Diploma as a Licentiate in Dental Surgery conferred by a university (LDS)
Diploma as a Licentiate awarded by the Royal Colleges
Licence in Dental Surgery of the Royal College of Surgeons of England

Licentiate in Dental Surgery of the Royal College of Surgeons of Edinburgh
Licentiate in Dental Surgery of the Royal College of Physicians and Surgeons of Glasgow.

Details of these awards are given in *British Qualifications* (Kogan Page) or may be obtained from the administering bodies.

Course for Dental Therapists/Hygienists

This is a two-year course of professional training which begins each September. Prospective students should be at least 17 by 1 September of the year in which they begin their studies and should have a minimum of five GCSE passes (or equivalent), including English and biology, chemistry and/or human biology. Relevant work experience is also required as a Dental Surgery Assistant with a DSA qualification.

Further information is available from the Dental Auxiliary School, Royal London Hospital Medical College, Turner Street London E1 2AD.

Higher Medical and Dental Qualifications

Higher qualifications for doctors and dentists divide into two groups: first, those awarded by examination by the various Royal Colleges which, for people wishing to work in hospital settings, are a necessity for promotion to independent status; second, higher degrees. In both cases, study is usually undertaken in a training post with the aid of a selection of short or part-time courses.

For details see *British Qualifications* (Kogan Page), or write to the awarding body concerned.

Postgraduate Awards

Medical Qualifications

Awards by Examination of the Royal Colleges
Royal College of General Practitioners
Associateship
Membership

Royal College of Obstetricians and Gynaecologists
Membership
Diploma

Royal College of Pathologists
Membership
Diploma in Clinical Cytogenetics and Molecular Genetics

Royal College of Physicians of Edinburgh
Membership
Diploma in Pharmaceutical Medicine
Diploma in Community Child Health
Diploma in Child Health
Diploma in Geriatric Medicine

Diploma in Medical Rehabilitation
Diploma in Tropical Medicine and Hygiene

Royal College of Physicians and Surgeons of Glasgow
Membership qua Physician
Fellowship qua Physician
Fellowship qua Surgeon

Royal College of Physicians of London
Membership

Royal Colleges of Physicians UK
Membership (in paediatrics and adult medicine)

Royal College of Psychiatrists
Membership

Royal College of Radiologists
Fellowship
Membership

Royal College of Surgeons in Edinburgh
Fellowship
Fellowship (Surgical Specialties): otolaryngology, gynaecological surgery, oral and maxillofacial surgery, ophthalmology, accident and emergency medicine and surgery

Royal College of Surgeons of England
Fellowship
There are subsidiary diplomas in two of the specialties with similar training requirements: the DO RCSEng and the DLO RSCEng (Parts I and II)
Fellowship of the College of Anaesthetics
Diploma in Anaesthetics

Other Postgraduate Awards in Medicine

The universities and Royal Colleges and other bodies confer degrees and diplomas in specialist areas of medicine, usually after full- or part-time courses of instruction.

Anaesthetics MSc (Med Sci) Anaesthesia: University of Glasgow: 2 yrs FT. MSc in Anaesthesia and Intensive Care: University of Wales College of Medicine: 2 yrs FT.

Anatomy MMedSc in Anatomy & Cell Biology: University of Sheffield: 1 yr. MMedSc in Ultrastructural Anatomy & Pathology: Queen's University Belfast: 1 yr FT.
MSc in Anatomical Science: University of Glasgow: 2 yrs FT.

Audiology MSc in Educational Audiology: University of Manchester: 1 yr FT. MSc in Audiological Medicine: University of London (University College): 1 yr FT; University of Manchester: 1 yr FT.

MSc in Audiology: University of Manchester: 1 yr FT (Department of Audiology and Education of the Deaf); University of Southampton: 1 yr FT or 6 mths FT plus research project undertaken externally over an equivalent period.
Diploma in Audiology: University of Southampton: 6 mths FT; University of Manchester: 1 yr FT.
Certificate in Audiology: University of Southampton: 6 mths FT.
MSc in Auditory Sciences: University of London (University College): 1 yr FT.

Bacteriology Diploma in Bacteriology: University of Manchester: 1 yr FT course.
MSc in Bacteriology: University of Manchester: 1 yr FT.
PhD in Bacteriology: University of Manchester: 3 yrs FT.
MMedSc in Bacteriology: Queen's University of Belfast: 1 yr FT 4 yrs PT.
MSc in Mineralised Tissue Biology: University of London (University College): 1 yr FT/2 yrs PT.

Biochemistry MSc in Clinical Biochemistry: University of Dublin, Trinity College: 3 yrs; University of Leeds: 1 yr FT; University of London (intercollegiate, organised by Charing Cross Hospital): 2 yrs PT; University of London (Royal Postgraduate Medical School): 2 yrs PT; University of Newcastle upon Tyne: 1 yr FT; University of Surrey: 1 yr FT/2 yrs block release.
MSc in Biochemistry: University of London (University College): 1 yr FT.
MSc in Analytical Biochemistry: University of Dundee: 1 yr FT.
MSc in Medical Biochemistry: Brunel University: PT/FT.
MSc in Biomedical Science Research: University of London (King's College): 1 yr FT/2 yrs PT.
Diploma in Bioanalytical Chemistry: University of Dundee: 9–12 mths FT.
MSc in Biosensors: University of Newcastle upon Tyne: 1 yr FT.

Cardiology MSc in Cardiovascular Studies: University of Leeds: 1 yr FT.
MSc (Med Sc) Medical Cardiology: University of Glasgow: 2 yrs FT.
Diploma in Cardiology: University of Leeds: 1 yr FT; University of London (National Heart & Lung Institute): 1 yr FT; University of London (Royal Postgraduate Medical School): 1 yr FT.

Clinical Cytology MSc in Clinical Cytotechnology: University of London (St Mary's Hospital Medical School): 1 yr FT 2 yrs PT.
Diploma in Gynaecological Cytotechnology: University of London (St Mary's Hospital Medical School): 6 mths.
MSc in Clinical Cytopathology: University of London Imperial College (St Mary's Hospital Medical School): 1 yr FT/2 yrs PT.

Dermatology MSc (MedSc) in Dermatology: University of Glasgow: 2 yrs FT.
Diploma in Dermatology: University of London (St John's Institute of Dermatology): 9 mths–1yr FT.
Diploma in Dermatological Sciences: University of Wales, College of Medicine: 1 yr FT.
Diploma in Practical Dermatology: University of Wales, College of Medicine: Distance learning.
MSc in Dermatology: University of Wales, College of Medicine: 1 yr.

MSc in Clinical Dermatology: University of London (St John's Institute of Dermatology): 1 yr FT; London University (United Medical and Dental Schools, Guy's and St Thomas's): 1 yr FT.

Endocrinology MSc/MMedSc in Endocrinology: University of Sheffield: 1 yr FT.
Diploma in Endocrinology: University of London (Royal Postgraduate Medical School): 1 yr FT.
MMedSc in Clinical and Molecular Endocrinology & Diabetes: University of Birmingham: 1 yr FT.
MSc in Neuroendocrine Cell Biology: University of London (University College & Royal Postgraduate Medical School): 1 yr FT.
MSc in Steroid Endocrinology: University of Leeds: 1 yr FT.

Epidemiology Diploma in Epidemiology: Royal College of Physicians: 1 yr FT.
MSc in Communicable Disease Epidemiology: University of Cambridge: 1 yr FT/2 yrs PT.
MSc in Environmental Epidemiology & Policy & Tropical Medicine: University of London (School of Hygiene & Tropical Medicine): 1 yr FT/2 yrs PT.
MSc in Epidemiology: University of London (School of Hygiene & Tropical Medicine): 1 yr FT/2 yrs PT.
MSc in Epidemiology and Health Planning: University of Wales (College of Swansea and College of Medicine): 1 yr FT.
MSc in Infectious Diseases: University of London (Royal Postgraduate Medical School): 1 yr FT.
MSc in Epidemiology and Biostatistics: Manchester University: 2 yrs PT.

Family Planning Certificate in Family Planning: Joint Committee on Contraception.
Certificate in Advanced Family Planning (including insertion of intra-uterine devices): Joint Committee on Contraception.

Forensic MSc in Forensic Science: University of London (King's College): 1 yr FT; University of Glasgow: 1 yr FT.
MSc or Diploma in Forensic Science: University of Strathclyde.
Diploma and Certificate in Forensic Medicine: University of Glasgow.
Diploma & MSc in Forensic Behavioural Science: University of Liverpool: 1 yr FT (diploma); 2 yrs PT (MSc).
Diploma in Forensic Psychiatry: University of London (Institute of Psychiatry): 1 yr FT/2 yrs PT.
Diploma in Forensic Toxicology: University of Glasgow: 1 yr.

General Medicine Diploma in Internal Medicine: University of London (Royal Postgraduate Medical School): 1 yr FT.
Diploma in Medical Science (DipMedSc) in Internal Medicine: University of Newcastle upon Tyne: 1 yr FT.
Master of Medical Science (MMedSc) in Internal Medicine: University of Newcastle upon Tyne: 1 yr FT.
MSc (MMedSc) in Internal Medicine: University of Glasgow: 2 yrs FT.

General Practice Diploma in Primary Medical Care: University of Keele: 2 yrs PT.
MSc in Primary Medical Care: University of Keele: 1 yr (additional to diploma).

MMedSc in General Practice: University of Birmingham: 2 yrs PT.
MSc in General Practice: University of London (United Medical Schools): 2 yrs PT.

General Surgery MMedSc of PhD: University of Birmingham.
Master of Surgery MCh: University of Bristol.
Master of Surgery MCh: University of Oxford.
MSc in Organ Transplantation: University of London (Royal Free Hospital): 1 yr FT.

Genetics MSc in Medical Genetics: University of Newcastle upon Tyne: 1 yr FT.
MSc (MedSc) in Medical Genetics: University of Glasgow: 1 yr FT.
Diploma in Clinical Genetics: University of London (Institute of Child Health): 9 mths FT.

Geriatric Medicine MSc/Diploma in Advanced Clinical Practice (Cancer Nursing/Care of the Elderly): University of Surrey: 2 yrs PT.
MSc (MedSc) in Geriatric Medicine: University of Glasgow: 2 yrs FT.
MSc in Gerontology: University of London (King's College): 2 yrs PT (FT possible); University of Liverpool: 2 yrs PT.
MSc Social Gerontology: University of Southampton.
MA in Gerontology: University of Wales (Bangor): 2 yrs PT.

Haematology MSc (MedSc) in Haematology: University of London (Royal Postgraduate Medical School): 1 yr FT; University of Glasgow: 2 yrs FT.

Immunology MSc in Immunology: University of Birmingham: 1 yr FT; University of London (Royal Postgraduate Medical School): 1 yr.
MSc in Clinical Immunology: University of Leeds: 1 yr FT.
MSc in Immunology of Infectious Diseases: University of London (School of Hygiene & Tropical Medicine): 1 yr FT.
MSc in Medical Genetics with Immunology: Brunel University: PT/FT.
MSc in Medical Immunology: University of London (United Medical Schools): 2 yrs FT; University of London (Imperial College): PT; University of London (King's College): 2 yrs PT.

Medical Demography MSc in Medical Demography: University of London (London School of Hygiene & Tropical Medicine): 1 yr FT/2 yrs PT.
Diploma in Medical Demography: as above: 1 yr FT.

Medical Education Diploma in Medical Education, University of Dundee: 1–4 yrs' distance learning; University of Wales, College of Medicine: 1 yr FT/2 yrs PT.
Master in Medical Education: University of Dundee: 1–4 yrs' distance learning (following diploma)/9 mths FT.
MSc and MPhil in Medical Education: University of Wales, College of Medicine: 1 yr FT/2 yrs PT.

Medical Jurisprudence MPhil in Medical Ethics & Law: University of Glasgow: 2 yrs FT.
MA Medical Ethics & Law: University of London (King's College): 1 yr FT/2 yrs PT; MPhil: Queen's University (Belfast): 2 yrs FT.

LLM in Legal Aspects of Medical Practice: University of Wales, College of Cardiff: 1 yr FT/2 yrs PT.
Diploma in Legal Medicine: University of Sheffield: 1 yr FT/2 yrs PT.

Medical Parasitology MSc in Medical Parasitology: University of London (London School of Hygiene & Tropical Medicine): 1 yr FT.
MSc/MVSc in Applied Parasitology and Medical Entomology: University of Liverpool: 1 yr FT.
MSc in Clinical Parasitology: University of London (Royal Free Hospital School of Medicine, London School of Hygiene & Tropical Medicine): 2 yrs PT.
MSc in Parasites and and Diseases: University of Wales (Bangor): 2 yrs FT.

Medical Physics and Biomedical Engineering MSc in Information Technology (Medical Physics): University of Aberdeen: 1 yr FT/2 yrs block release.
Diploma in Information Technology (Medical Physics): University of Aberdeen: 9 mths.
MSc in Medical Physics: University of Aberdeen: 1 yr FT; University of Leeds: 1 yr FT; University of Exeter: 1 yr FT.
Diploma in Medical Physics: University of Aberdeen: 9 mths FT.
MSc in Radiation Physics: University of London (intercollegiate): 1 yr FT.
Diploma in Biomedical Methods: University of Wales (College of Medicine): 1 yr PT.
Postgraduate Diploma in Biomechanics: University of Strathclyde: 9 mths (by distance learning).
MSc in Biophysics and Medical Physics: University of London (Birkbeck College): 2 yrs PT.
MMedSc in Biomedical Ethics: University of Birmingham: 1 yr PT.
MSc in Biomedical Engineering: University of Aberdeen: 1 yr FT/2 yrs block release.
Diploma in Biomedical Engineering: University of Aberdeen: 9 mths; University of Dundee: 9 mths FT.
MSc in Biomedical Engineering Science: University of Dundee: 1 yr FT.
MSc/Diploma in Biomedical Engineering: University of Surrey: 1 yr FT.
MSc in Biomedical Instrumentation: University of Dundee: 1 yr FT.
MSc in Physical Sciences in Medicine: University of Dublin: 3 yrs PT.
MSc in Biomedical Engineering Science: University of Dundee: 1 yr FT.
MSc Engineering & Physical Science in Medicine: University of London (Imperial College): 1 yr FT.
MSc/Diploma in Bioengineering: University of Strathclyde: 1 yr FT/2 yrs PT.
MSc in Medical Engineering & Physics: University of London (intercollegiate, organised by King's College): 2 yrs PT.
MSc in Biomedical Engineering and Medical Physics: University of Keele: 2 yrs PT.

Medical Statistics and Data Management MSc in Applied Stochastic Systems: University of London (University College): 1 yr FT/2 yrs PT.
MSc in Health Informatics: University of Glasgow: 1 yr FT.
MSc in Medical Statistics: University of London (London School of Hygiene & Tropical Medicine): 1 yr FT.
MSc/Diploma in Medical Statistics: University of Newcastle upon Tyne: 1 yr FT.

Microbiology MSc in Medical Microbiology: University of London (London School of Hygiene & Tropical Medicine): 1 yr FT.
MSc/Diploma in Medical Microbiology: University of Surrey: 2 yrs PT.
MSc/Diploma in General & Medical Microbiology: University of London (University College, School of Hygiene & Tropical Medicine): 1 yr FT.
MSc in Medical Biochemistry: University of Newcastle upon Tyne: 1 yr FT.
MSc/Diploma in Clinical Microbiology: University of London (London Hospital): 2 yrs PT.
MSc in Medical Microbiology (PhD also available): University of Manchester: 15 mths FT/9 mths FT + 6 mths research.

Molecular Biology MSc in Applied Molecular Biology & Biotechnology: University of London (University College): 1 yr FT.
MSc in Applied Molecular Biology of Infectious Diseases: University of London (London School of Hygiene & Tropical Medicine): 1 yr FT.
MSc in Molecular Microbiology: University of Manchester: 1 yr FT.

Nephrology Diploma in Nephrology and Hypertension: University of London (Royal Postgraduate Medical School): 1 yr FT.

Neuroscience/Neurology MSc in Speech & Language Pathology & Therapy: University of London (Institute of Neurology): 2½ yrs FT.
MSc in Neuroendocrine Cell Biology: University of London (University College & Royal Postgraduate Medical School): 1 yr FT.
MSc in Neurological Science: University of London (University College): 1 yr FT.
MSc in Neuroscience: University of London (Institute of Psychiatry/Ophthalmology): 1 yr FT.
MSc in Human Communication: University of London (Institute of Neurology): 1 yr FT/2 yrs PT.
Diploma in Clinical Neurology: University of London (Institute of Neurology): 6 mths.
MSc in Clinical Neurology: University of Oxford: 2 yrs FT.

Nuclear Medicine MSc in Nuclear Medicine: University of London (London Hospital): 1 yr FT/PT; University of London (Institute of Nuclear Medicine): 1 yr FT/PT; University of London (Royal Postgraduate Medical School): 1 yr FT/2 yrs PT; University of London (United Medical and Dental Schools, Guy's & St Thomas's)
MSc in Radiation Biology: University of London (intercollegiate, organised by University College): 1 yr FT/2 yrs PT.

Nutrition MSc/Diploma in Human Nutrition & Metabolism: University of Aberdeen: 1 yr FT; diploma 9 mths FT.
MSc in Nutrition: University of London (King's College): 1 yr FT.
MSc in Human Nutrition: University of London (London School of Hygiene & Tropical Medicine): 1 yr FT.
MMedSci in Human Nutrition: University of Sheffield: 1 yr FT.
Diploma in Human Nutrition: University of Aberdeen: 9 mths.

Obstetrics and Gynaecology Diploma in Obstetrics & Gynaecology (DGO): University of Dublin.

Licentiate in Midwifery (LM): University of Dublin.
Master of Obstetrics & Gynaecology (MObstG): University of Liverpool: 19 mths FT.
MSc/Diploma in Advanced Midwifery Practice: University of Surrey & Royal College of Midwives: 1 yr FT + 1 yr PT.
MSc in Reproductive Biology: University of Edinburgh: 1 yr FT.
MSc in Human Reproductive Biology: University of London (Royal Postgraduate Medical School): 1 yr FT.
MMedSci in Assisted Reproduction Technology: University of Nottingham: 1 yr FT.
Diploma in Obstetrics & Gynaecology: University of London (Royal Postgraduate Medical School; Institute of Gynaecology): 5½ mths FT.

Occupational Medicine Certificate in Aviation Medicine (Cert A Med): Faculty of Occupational Medicine, Royal College of Physicians – RAF Institute of Aviation Medicine: 4 two-week courses.
Certificate in Occupational Health: University of Aberdeen & Institute of Occupational Medicine Ltd, Edinburgh: 10 weeks FT.
Certificate in Occupational Hygiene: University of Aberdeen & Institute of Occupational Medicine Ltd, Edinburgh: 10 weeks FT.
Certificate in Underwater Medicine: University of Aberdeen: 3 yrs (modular).
Diploma in Aviation Medicine (DipAvMed): Faculty of Occupational Medicine, Royal College of Physicians – RAF Institute of Aviation Medicine: 6 mths.
Diploma in Occupational Health (DipOccH): University College Dublin: 2 yrs PT.
Diploma in Occupational Therapy: University of London (London Hospital Medical College): 25 mths FT.
MSc in Ergonomics: University of Aberdeen & Institute of Occupational Medicine, Edinburgh: 1 yr FT.
MSc in Occupational Health: University of Aberdeen & Institute of Occupational Medicine, Edinburgh: 1 yr FT/2 yrs PT.
MSc/Advanced Diploma in Occupational Health: University of Surrey: modular course.
MSc in Occupational Health Sciences: University of Manchester: 1 yr FT/2 yrs PT.
MSc in Occupational Hygiene: University of Aberdeen & Institute of Occupational Medicine, Edinburgh: 1 yr FT/2 yrs PT; University of Newcastle upon Tyne: 1 yr FT.
MSc/Advanced Diploma in Occupational Safety: University of Surrey: modular with research and dissertation/Modular credit accumulation.
MMedSci in Occupational Medicine: University of Birmingham: 1 yr FT.
MA in Health Services Management: University of Manchester: 9 mths FT.
MSc/Advanced Diploma in Occupational and Organisational Psychology: University of Surrey: 2 yrs FT: 1yr FT/2 yrs PT.

Ophthalmology FRCS: University of Aberdeen: 1 yr FT.
MSc in Ophthalmology: University of Glasgow (Tennant Institute of Ophthalmology): 2 yrs FT.
MSc in Community Eye Health: University of London (Institute of Ophthalmology): 1 yr FT.
Diploma in Community Eye Health: University of London (Institute of Ophthalmology): 6 mths.

MSc in Ophthalmology: University of Bristol, Bristol Eye Hospital: 1 academic yr plus a period of research for dissertation.
MSc (MedSc) in Ophthalmology: University of Glasgow: 2 yrs FT.
Certificate in Community Eye Health: University of London (Institute of Ophthalmology): 2 mths.
Certificate in Tropical Ophthalmology: University of London (Institute of Ophthalmology): 2 mths.

Orthopaedics Master of Orthopaedic Surgery (MChOrth): University of Liverpool: 1 yr FT.
MSc in Orthopaedics: University of London (University College): 1 yr FT/2 yrs PT; University of London (Institute of Orthopaedics): 1 yr.

Oto-Laryngology MSc (MedSc) in Oto-Laryngology: University of Glasgow: 2 yrs FT.

Paediatrics Certificate in Community Paediatrics for GPs: University of Sheffield: 1 yr PT.
Diploma in Child Health: University of Dublin: 6 wks PT.
Diploma in Community Paediatrics: University of Sheffield: 1 yr PT; University of Warwick: 2 yrs PT.
Diploma in Child & Adolescent Psychiatry: University of London (Institute of Child Health/Psychiatry) 1 yr FT.
Diploma in Clinical Genetics: University of London (Institute of Child Health): 9 mths FT.
Diploma in Community Based Rehabilitation: University of London (Institute of Child Health).
Diploma in Clinical Paediatrics: University of London (Institute of Child Health): 1 yr FT.
Diploma in Tropical Child Health (DTCH): University of Liverpool (Liverpool School of Tropical Medicine & Dept of Child Health): 6 mths FT.
Diploma in Paediatric Surgery: University of London (Institute of Child Health): 1 yr FT.
MSc in Community Paediatrics: University of London (Institute of Child Health); University of Newcastle upon Tyne: 2 yrs PT; University of Warwick: 1 yr FT/4 yrs PT.
MSc in Mother and Child Health: University of London (Institute of Child Health).
Master in Tropical Paediatrics (MTropPaed): University of Liverpool (Liverpool School of Tropical Medicine & Dept of Child Health): 1 yr FT.
Master in Clinical Genetics: University of London (Institute of Child Health): 1 yr FT.

Pathology Diplomas in Clinical & Chemical Pathology (DCP): University of London (Royal Postgraduate Medical School): 1 yr FT.
MSc in Experimental Pathology (Toxicology): University of London (Royal Postgraduate Medical School): 1 yr FT.
MMedSc in Clinical Pathology: University of Sheffield: 1 yr FT.
MMedSc in Pathology: Queen's University, Belfast: 2 yrs FT.
MMedSc in Ultrastructural Anatomy & Pathology: Queen's University, Belfast: 1 yr FT.
MSc (Med Sc) in Diagnostic Histopathology: University of Glasgow: 2 yrs FT.

Pharmacology/Pharmacy MSc in Pharmaceutical Analysis: University of Strathclyde: 1/2 yrs FT.
MSc in Pharmaceutical Services & Medicines Control: University of Bradford: 1 yr FT.
MSc in Pharmaceutical Technology: University of London (King's College): 1 yr FT/2 yrs PT.
MSc in Pharmaceutical & Quality Control: University of London (King's College): 1 yr FT/2 yrs PT.
MSc in Biopharmacy: University of London (King's College): 1 yr FT/2 yrs PT.
Diploma in Pharmaceutical Analysis: University of Strathclyde: 1 yr FT.
Diploma in Clinical Science: University of Wales (College of Cardiff & Welsh School of Pharmacy): 2 yrs PT.
Diploma in Clinical Pharmacy: University of Wales (College of Cardiff & Welsh School of Pharmacy): 2 yrs PT.
MSc in Clinical Pharmacy: University of Strathclyde: 1–2 yrs FT/2 yrs PT.
MSc (MedSc) in Clinical Pharmacology: University of Glasgow: 1–2 yrs FT.
MSc in Clinical Pharmacology: University of Aberdeen: 1 yr FT.
MSc in Pharmacology: University of Manchester: 1–2 yrs FT; University of Strathclyde: 1–2 yrs FT.
Postgraduate Diploma in Pharmacology: University of Strathclyde: 1 yr FT.
MSc in Biochemical Pharmacology: University of Southampton: 1 yr FT.
MSc or Postgraduate Diploma in Clinical Pharmacology: University of Aberdeen: 1 yr FT.
Diploma in Radiopharmaceutical Sciences: University of London (King's College): 2 yrs PT.
MSc in Experimental Drug Research: University of London (King's College): 2 yrs PT.
MSc in Pharmacology: University of London (King's College): 1 yr FT.
Postdoctoral Diploma in Pharmaceutical Sciences: University of London (King's College): 1 yr FT.
Postgraduate Diploma in Clinical Pharmacology: University of Aberdeen: 1 yr FT.
Diploma in Pharmacology: University of Manchester: 2 yrs PT/1 yr FT.

Psychiatry MMedSci in Clinical Psychiatry: University of Leeds: 3 yrs PT.
MSc in Psychiatry: University of Manchester: 3 yrs PT; University of London (Institute of Psychiatry): 2 yrs PT; University of Cambridge: 3 yrs PT; University of Dundee: 2 yrs PT; University of Keele: 2 yrs PT.
MPhil in Psychiatry: University of Edinburgh: 3 yrs PT; University of London (Institute of Psychiatry): 3 yrs; University of London (Imperial College) 3 yrs PT.
Diploma in Psychiatry: University of Edinburgh: 2 yrs PT; University of Manchester: 2 yrs PT.
Diploma in Child and Adolescent Psychiatry: University of London (Institute of Child Health/Psychiatry): 1 yr FT.
Diploma in Forensic Psychiatry: University of London (Institute of Psychiatry): 1 yr FT/2 yrs PT.
MMedSc in Psychiatry: University of Birmingham: 3 yrs PT.
Board Certification in Psychiatry: University of London (Institute of Psychiatry).
Diploma in Addiction: University of London (Institute of Psychiatry): 1 yr.

MSc/Diploma in General Psychiatry: University of Keele: 1 yr PT (diploma); 2 yrs PT (MSc).
Diploma in Child and Adolescent Psychiatry: University of London (Institute of Psychiatry and Institute of Health) 1 yr FT.
MSc in Advanced Mental Health Studies: University of Dundee: 1 yr FT/2 yrs PT.

Public Health Medicine (including Community Medicine) Certificate in Health & the Family in Developing Countries: University of Wales, College of Medicine: 3 mths.
Certificate in Health Care: Professions allied to medicine: University of Exeter.
Certificate in Marketing for Health Care & Public Services: University of Leeds (Nuffield Institute for Health Service Studies): 8–9 mths PT.
Certificate/Diploma/MSc in Public Health: University of Aberdeen: 4 mths FT (certificate); 9 mths FT (diploma); 1 yr FT (MSc).
Diploma in Advanced Study in Education for Primary Health Care: University of Manchester: 9 mths FT/2 yrs PT.
Diploma in Business Administration (Health, Population & Nutrition in Developing Countries): University of Keele: 9 mths FT.
Diploma in Community Health Care: University of the South Bank: 1 yr FT.
Diploma in Community Eye Health: University of London (Institute of Ophthalmology): 6 mths.
Diploma in Community Health: University of Edinburgh: 9 mths FT/21 mths PT.
Diploma in Environmental Health: University of Edinburgh: 9 mths FT/21 mths PT.
Diploma in Community Health Care Studies: Wales (Swansea): 1 yr FT.
Diploma in Health Management, Planning & Policy: University of Leeds (Nuffield Institute of Health Service Studies): 1 yr FT.
Diploma in Health Medicine: University of Cambridge: 1 yr FT.
Diploma in Health Promotion & Health Education: University of Edinburgh: 9 mths FT/21 mths PT.
Diploma in Health Sciences: University of Edinburgh: 9 mths FT/21 mths PT.
Diploma in Hospital Management: University of Leeds (Nuffield Institute of Health Service Studies): 1 yr FT.
Diploma in Management (for Doctors): University of Keele: 18 mths PT.
Diploma/MSc in Health Education & Health Promotion: University of Leeds (Nuffield Institute of Health Service Studies).
Diploma/MSc in Hospital or Primary Health Care Management for Developing Countries: University of Birmingham: 9 mths FT (diploma); 1 yr FT (MSc).
MA in Health Services Studies: University of Leeds (Nuffield Institute of Health Service Studies): 1 yr FT/2 yrs PT.
MA in Community and Health Ethics: University of Central Lancashire: 2 yrs PT.
MSc in Community Medicine: University of Newcastle: 2 yrs PT.
MA in Community Care (Learning Disability): University of Keele: 1 yr FT.
MA in Quality Assurance in Health & Social Care: University of Leeds (Nuffield Institute of Health Service Studies): 20 mths.
Master in Community Health (MCommH): University of Liverpool (School of Tropical Medicine): 1 yr FT.
Master in Health Management: City University, London: 2 yrs PT.

MBA (Health & Social Services option): University of Leeds (Nuffield Institute of Health Service Studies): 24–36 mths.
MBA (Health Executive Programme): University of Keele: 2 yrs PT.
MBA (Health, Population & Nutrition in Developing Countries): University of Keele: 1 yr FT.
MMedSci in Primary & Community Care: University of Sheffield: 1 yr FT.
MPH: University College, Dublin: 1 yr FT/2 yrs PT; University of Dundee: 1 yr FT; University of Glasgow: 1 yr FT/2 yrs PT; University of Leeds: 1 yr FT; University of Liverpool: 1 yr FT; University of Wales, College of Medicine: 1 yr FT.
MPH for Warm Climate Countries: University of Leeds (Nuffield Institute of Health Service Studies): 1 yr FT.
MSc in Communicable Disease Epidemiology: University of London (School of Hygiene & Tropical Medicine): 1 yr FT.
MSc in Community Health: University of Dublin (Trinity College): 1 yr FT; University of Edinburgh: 1 yr FT/2 yrs PT.
MSc in Community Health in Developing Countries: University of London (School of Hygiene & Tropical Medicine): 1 yr FT.
MSc in Community Medicine: University of Manchester: 2 yrs PT.
MSc in Environmental Health: University of Dundee: 1 yr FT; University of Edinburgh: 1 yr FT/2 yrs PT.
MSc in Environmental Health (Water Quality Management): University of Surrey: 6½ mths FT.
MSc in Epidemiology and Health Planning: University of Wales (College of Swansea/Medicine): 1 yr FT.
MSc in Health Care: University of Exeter.
MSc in Health Care: Professional Education: University of Exeter.
MSc in Health Informatics: University of Glasgow: 1 yr.
MSc in Health Planning and Financing: University of London (LSE & School of Hygiene & Tropical Medicine): 1 yr FT/2 yrs PT.
MSc in Health Promotion: University of London (School of Hygiene & Tropical Medicine): 1 yr FT/2 yrs PT.
MSc in Health Promotion and Health Education: University of Edinburgh: 1 yr FT/2 yrs PT.
MSc in Public Health Engineering: University of Leeds: 1 yr FT/2 yrs PT.
MSc in Health Sciences: University of Edinburgh: 1 yr FT/2 yrs PT; University of London (St George's Hospital): 2 yrs PT.
MSc in Health Services Management: University of London (School of Hygiene & Tropical Medicine): 1 yr FT.
MSc in Preventative Health Care for Developing Countries: University of Wales: College of Medicine: 1 yr FT.
MSc in Public Health: University of Aberdeen: 1 yr FT; University of Dundee: 1 yr FT; University of Glasgow: 1 yr FT; University of Leeds: 1 yr FT; University of Manchester: 1 yr FT.
MSc in Public Health in Developing Countries: University of London (School of Hygiene & Tropical Medicine): 1 yr FT.
MSc in Public Health Medicine: University of London (School of Hygiene & Tropical Medicine): 1 yr FT/2 yrs PT; University of Newcastle upon Tyne: 2 yrs PT.
MSc/Postgraduate Diploma in Environmental Management & Health: University of Surrey.

MSc in Community Paediatrics: University of Newcastle: 2 yrs PT; University of Nottingham: 2 yrs PT.
Postgraduate Diploma in Quality Assurance In Health & Social Care: University of Leeds (Nuffield Institute of Health Service Studies): 15 mths.
Postgraduate Diploma/MA in Health Management, Planning & Policy: University of Leeds (Nuffield Institute of Health Service Studies): 1 yr FT.
Postgraduate Diploma/MSc in Health Service Management: South Bank University: 3 trms (diploma); 4 trms (MSc).

Radiotherapeutics and Clinical Oncology Diploma/MSc in Clinical Oncology: University of Edinburgh: 2 yrs FT.
MSc in Radiotherapy and Oncology: University of Dundee: 2 yrs PT.
Diploma in Clinical Oncology: University of London (Institute of Cancer Research): 9 mths.
MSc in Cancer Sciences: University of London (University College): 2 yrs PT.
MSc (MedSc) in Oncology: University of Glasgow: 2 yrs PT; University of Manchester: 2 yrs PT.

Rehabilitation Certificate in Rehabilitation Engineering: University of London (King's College): 1 yr PT.
Diploma in Rehabilitation Engineering: University of London (King's College): 1 yr PT.
MSc in Rehabilitation Management: University of Newcastle: 2 yrs PT.
Diploma in Rehabilitation Technology: University of Dundee: 9 mths FT.
MSc in Rehabilitation Studies: University of Southampton: 2 yrs PT.
MSc in Rehabilitation Counselling: Institute of West London: 2 yrs PT.

Rheumatology MMedSc in Rheumatology: University of Birmingham: 1 yr FT.
MSc in Rheumatology: University of Manchester: 2 yrs PT.

Sociology of Medicine MSc Sociology as applied to Medicine: University of London (Royal Holloway College): 1 yr FT.
MSc in Sociology (Health and Illness): University of the South Bank: 2 yrs PT.

Sports Medicine Diploma in Sports Medicine: University of London (London Hospital): 24 wks FT; University of Dublin (Trinity College): 1 yr FT.
MMedSc in Sport & Exercise Science: University of Sheffield: 1 yr FT.
Certificate & Diploma in Sports Physiotherapy: Association of Chartered Physiotherapists in Sports Medicine, Crewe & Alsager College of Higher Education: 6 mths (certificate); 2 yrs PT (diploma).
MPhil in Sports Medicine: University of London British Postgraduate Medical Foundation.
MSc in Sport and Exercise Sciences: University of Ulster: 2 yrs PT.
MSc in Sports Medicine: University of Nottingham: 2 yrs PT.
MSc in the Science of Sports Coaching: University of Sheffield: 1 yr FT.
MSc in Sports Sciences: University of Loughborough: 1 yr FT/2 yrs PT.

Thoracic Medicine Diploma in Thoracic Medicine: University of London (National Heart & Lung Institute): 1 yr FT.
Diploma in Tuberculosis and Chest Diseases: University of Wales, College of Medicine: 6 mths FT.

MSc in Thoracic Medicine: University of London (National Heart & Lung Institute): 1–2 yrs FT.

Toxicology MSc in Applied Toxicology: University of Surrey: 3–7 yrs PT; University of Portsmouth: 2 yrs PT.
MSc in Toxicology: University of Surrey: 1 yr FT/2 yrs PT.
MSc/Diploma in Toxicology: University of Birmingham: 1 yr.
Postgraduate Diploma in Toxicology: University of Surrey: 1 yr FT/2 yrs PT.
Diploma in Toxicology: University of Dublin (Trinity College): 2 yrs PT.

Tropical Medicine and Hygiene Diploma in Tropical Medicine and Hygiene (DTM&H): Royal College of Physicians (London School of Hygiene & Tropical Medicine): 3 mths FT; University of Liverpool: 3 mths FT.
Diploma in Tropical Child Health (DTCH): University of Liverpool (Liverpool School of Tropical Medicine): 6 mths FT.
MSc in Tropical Medicine: University of Liverpool (Liverpool School of Tropical Medicine): 2 yrs FT.
Master of Tropical Medicine (MTropMed): University of Liverpool (Liverpool School of Tropical Medicine): 1 yr FT.
Master in Tropical Paediatrics (MTropPaed): University of Liverpool (Liverpool School of Tropical Medicine): 1 yr FT.
MSc in Tropical Paediatrics: University of Liverpool: 2 yrs PT.
MSc in Infection & Health in the Tropics: University of London (School of Hygiene & Tropical Medicine): 1 yr FT.
MSc in Medical Entomology: University of London (School of Hygiene & Tropical Medicine): 12 mths FT.

Urology Diploma in Urology: University of London (Institute of Urology & Nephrology): 1 yr FT.

Vascular Medicine MSc Vascular Medicine & Technology: University of London (St Mary's Hospital): 1 yr FT/2 yrs PT.

Venereology Diploma in Venereology: University of Liverpool: 3 mths FT.

Virology MSc in Virology: University of London (London School of Hygiene & Tropical Medicine): 1 yr FT.
MSc in Medical Virology: University of London (Royal Free Hospital School of Medicine & London School of Hygiene & Tropical Medicine): 2 yrs PT (day release); University of Manchester: 1 yr FT.

Dental Qualifications

Awards by Examination of the Royal Colleges
Royal College of Surgeons of Edinburgh
Fellowship in Dental Surgery
Licentiate in Dental Surgery
Diploma in Restorative Dentistry

Royal College of Surgeons of England
Diploma in Dental Surgery
Diploma in Dental Public Health

Diploma in Orthodontics
Membership in General Dental Surgery

Royal College of Physicians and Surgeons of Glasgow
Licentiate in Dental Surgery
Membership in General Dental Surgery
Membership in Clinical Community Dentistry

University Higher Degrees and Diplomas
All universities which confer a first degree award the higher degree of Master of Dental Surgery (MDS) or Dental Science (MDSc). Some universities also award a doctorate.

Master of Dental Surgery (MDS) or Dental Science (MDSc) degrees are awarded by the following universities: Abertay, Belfast, Birmingham, Bristol, Dundee, Glasgow, Leeds, Liverpool, London, Manchester, Newcastle, Sheffield, Wales and Dublin.

Doctor of Dental Surgery (DDS) and Doctor of Dental Science (DDSc) degrees are awarded by the following universities: Abertay, Birmingham, Dundee, Glasgow, Leeds, Manchester, Newcastle, Wales.

It is also possible to take other higher degrees at universities (MPhil, MSc and PhD) in relevant fields of study.

Courses in Complementary and Alternative Medicine

Below are listed some of the courses approved by professional associations of the disciplines outlined in this book which qualify students for inclusion on their register of practitioners. Tuition fees are payable for all courses and grants are rarely available. Most courses are, however, part time, thus enabling students to continue working during their studies. Further information can be obtained from the addresses below.

Acupuncture

As from October 1995 there is one UK governing body, the British Acupuncture Council, Park House, 206–208 Latimer Road, London W10 6XY. The British Acupuncture Accreditation Board sets and monitors standards in acupuncture training with the aim of ensuring accreditation of competent acupuncture schools. So far, five colleges have been accorded candidacy status with a view to eventual accreditation: the British College of Acupuncture, 8 Hunter Street, London WC1N 1BN; the College of Traditional Acupuncture UK, Tao House, Queensway, Royal Leamington Spa, Warwickshire CV31 3LZ; the International College of Oriental Medicine UK, Green Hedges House, Green Hedges Avenue, East Grinstead, West Sussex RH19 1DZ; the London School of Acupuncture and Traditional Chinese Medicine, Fourth Floor, 60 Bunhill Row, London EC1Y 8DQ; and the Northern College of Acupuncture, 124 Acomb Road, York YO2 4EY.

Alexander Technique

The Society of Teachers of the Alexander Technique (STAT), 20 London House, 266 Fulham Road, London SW10 9EL
This is the umbrella organisation for people teaching the Alexander technique.

A three-year teacher training course is offered at a number of training schools which are recognised and approved by STAT. A programme of continuous assessment leads to a Certificate in Professional Competence from the school and full membership of the Society. Application should be made to the head of the training course chosen, details of which can be obtained from STAT, and admission is solely at the discretion of the head of the college.

Healing

National Federation of Spiritual Healers, Old Manor Farm Studio, Church Street, Sunbury-on-Thames, Middlesex TW16 6RG
This is the umbrella organisation for healers in the UK. For details about healing contact the address above.

Herbal Medicine

National Institute of Medical Herbalists, 56 Longbrook Street, Exeter, Devon EX4 6AH
Membership is by examination after completing a four-year course of training. All members are required to adhere to a strict professional code of ethics demanded by the Institute and to carry the letters of qualification after their name, either MNIMH or FNIMH (Master or Fellow). The Institute runs a four-year BSc degree course in Herbal Medicine in London at Middlesex University.

School of Phytotherapy (Herbal Medicine), Bucksteep Manor, Bodle Street Green, Hailsham, East Sussex BN27 4RJ
The curriculum of the School covers the full range of medical and botanical sciences. A number of courses are offered. There is a four-year full-time degree course, validated by the University of Wales and covering three years of theoretical and practical tuition and a fourth year of specialist clinical training. As well as providing a comprehensive training in herbal medicine the course includes an analysis of the principles and philosophy of medical herbalism, an investigation of the constituents and pharmacology of medicinal plants, a study of the human body in health and disease, as well as practical training in diagnostic and therapeutic techniques. A Diploma in Phytotherapy is awarded on successful completion of an exam after the fourth year of study. There is also a four-year part-time home-based tutorial course, comprising 500 hours of clinical training, practical study and tutorial work. Home study averages 20–30 hours a week, depending on the student's ability and rate of work. A Certificate in Herbal Medicine is awarded on successful completion of an exam at the end of the fourth year. There is a one-year home-based training course in herbal medicine, designed for the lay-person who has an interest in plant remedies. The aim is to provide a basic understanding of the human body and to give the student a working knowledge of the use of British indigenous herbs in the treatment of non-severe ailments. An optional exam is available at the end of the course leading to a Certificate in Herbal Studies. It must be noted that this qualification does not constitute a licence to practise professionally.

Homoeopathy

The Society of Homoeopaths, 2 Artizan Road, Northampton NN1 4HU
The Society maintains a Register of practising homoeopaths of skill and repute. It does not offer any regular courses but does organise seminars and conferences for its members. Colleges recommended by the Society are listed below. The courses they run are usually four years in duration with the emphasis in the

first three years being on theory and with the fourth year being geared more towards practice. The colleges usually run courses on long weekends throughout the year, although in the fourth year sessions are run mid-week and are held in college clinics. For details of the courses at the following organisations, please apply direct to the Registrar of the college concerned:

British School of Homoeopathy, Pump Cottage, Compton, Durville, South Petherton, Somerset TA13 5ER; *Purton House School of Homoeopathy*, Purton House, Purton Lane, Farnham Royal, Buckinghamshire SL2 3LY; *The London College of Classical Homoeopathy*, Morely College, 61 Westminster Bridge Road, London SE1 7HT; *The College of Practical Homoeopathy*, 186 Wolverhampton Street, Dudley, West Midlands DY1 3AD; *The Northern College of Homoeopathic Medicine*, First Floor, Swinburne House, Swinburne Street, Gateshead, Tyne and Wear NE8 1AX; *The School of Homoeopathic Medicine*, 46 London Meadow Road, Alfreton, Derbyshire DE55 7PD; *The Yorkshire School of Homoeopathy*, Lansdown, 24 Rosebank, Burley-in-Wharfedale, Ilkley, West Yorkshire LS29 7RQ; *North West College of Homoeopathy*, 23 Wilbraham Road, Fallowfield, Manchester M14 6FB; *The College of Classical Homoeopathy*, Othergates Clinic, 45 Barrington Street, Tiverton, Devon EX16 6QP; *The School of Homoeopathy*, Yondercott House, Uffculme, Devon EX15 3DR; *The Scottish College of Homoeopathy*, Lynedock Place, Glasgow, Strathclyde G3 6AB; *The School for Advanced Homoeopathic Studies*, 69 West Malvern Road, West Malvern, Worcestershire WR14 4NP.

Hypnotherapy

National Association of Counsellors, Hypnotherapists and Psychotherapists, (The Director of Studies, NACHP Training Faculty, 145 Coleridge Road, Cambridge CB1 3PN), is a professional association of qualified therapists which has five grades of membership: Student Membership, Associate Membership, Full Membership, Subscribing Membership and Fellowship. There is a course which is designed to provide a thorough background and knowledge of counselling skills, hypnosis and psychotherapy. It should appeal both to those who have an interest in their own growth and development, as well as to those who intend to make hypnotherapy and psychotherapy their career. The course is also suitable for people working within the caring professions who wish to use the therapies as an adjunct to their present work.

Students must be at least 25 years old, and have achieved the minimum standard university entrance requirements of five GCSEs and five A levels. Mature candidates who are unable to fulfil these criteria are asked to demonstrate their ability and commitment to undertake the course.

The course aims to give prospective therapists a thorough background in all the skills they are likely to need to work with the client as an individual in a non-judgmental, empathic and eclectic way. This includes counselling skills, hypnosis and its therapeutic applications, psychotherapy, psychology, basic anatomy and physiology, neuro-linguistic programming and practice management.

National College of Hypnosis and Psychotherapy, 12 Cross Street, Nelson, Lancashire BB9 7EN, offers training in hypnotherapy and psychotherapy through part-time courses, held at weekends, in London, Cheshire and Glasgow. It is the first college of its kind to be externally accredited by the British Accreditation Council for Independent Further and Higher Education, following rigorous inspection of all aspects of the College's operation. The training is in three stages: Stage One, the foundation course, aims to give students a knowledge of hypnosis and to train them to be efficient in inducing the hypnotic states, and in its management, with the emphasis on practical training; Stage Two covers theories of psychotherapy and additional techniques in hypnotherapy, and successful completion of this stage, based on assessed coursework and examination, leads to the award of the Certificate in Hypnotherapy and Psychotherapy; Stage Three leads to the award of the Diploma in Hypnotherapy and Psychotherapy upon successful completion of a dissertation and a practical examination. All courses are led by experienced, practising therapists.

Osteopathy

The General Council and Register of Osteopaths (GCRO), 56 London Street, Reading, Berkshire RG1 4SQ

The organisation establishes and maintains standards of osteopathic education, and establishes and maintains standards of professional and ethical behaviour of its members. Four schools provide accredited courses which are regularly inspected by the GCRO. They are: *The British College of Naturopathy and Osteopathy (BCNO)*, Frazer House, 6 Netherhall Gardens, London NW3 5RR; *The British School of Osteopathy (BSO)*, 1–4 Suffolk Street, London SW1Y 4HG; *The European School of Osteopathy (ESO)*, 104 Tonbridge Road, Maidstone, Kent ME16 8SL; and *The London College of Osteopathic Medicine (LCOM)*, 8–10 Boston Place, London NW1 6QH. The BCNO and BSO offer four-year full-time degree courses. The LCOM runs a 13-month course for qualified doctors (physicians). All the accredited courses contain a mixture of theoretical sciences, practical work and clinical work with patients. Graduates from the four courses are eligible for membership of the GCRO.

The British College of Naturopathy and Osteopathy (address above) runs a four-year BSc (Hons) in Osteopathic Medicine. Candidates must be at least 18 years of age and have two A levels in chemistry and biological science, together with three GCSE passes, including English. Mature students may be considered on an individual basis. All applicants must show they have adequate financial resources to complete the course. Subjects studied are: biology, anatomy, physiology, pathology, osteopathic technique, neuro-muscular technique, nutrition, principles and philosophy of natural therapeutics, principles and philosophy of osteopathy, soft-tissue techniques, psychology, clinical subjects, orthopaedics and traumatology, clinical dietetics, clinical osteopathy, clinical practice, applied natural therapeutics, diagnosis, osteopathic diagnosis, laboratory techniques, x-ray diagnosis, gynaecology, paediatrics and pharmacology.

Further information about osteopathy can be obtained from the Osteopathic Information Service, PO Box 2074, Reading, Berkshire RG1 4YR.

Professional Training in Mental Health

Psychology

The British Psychological Society (BPS), St Andrews House, 48 Princess Road East, Leicester LE1 7DR maintains a Register of Chartered Psychologists.

Whatever first degree course you choose in psychology, you are advised to make sure that it is accredited by the BPS as conferring the Graduate Basis for

Registration (GBR). The GBR is a prerequisite to postgraduate training in psychology and may be considered as the preliminary qualification for the practice of psychology in the UK. It is the first step towards registration as a Chartered Psychologist. If, however, you are currently enrolled on, or have completed, a degree which is not accredited as conferring GBR, you can achieve this by taking a further qualification which has been accredited. This does not need to be a full degree and may be a conversion course which may take a year or two to complete and may be taken either full or part time. Alternatively, graduates with non accredited degrees may wish to undertake the Society's Qualifying Examination.

Examinations

Qualifying Examination of the Society: Candidates must hold a degree from a recognised university or other institution. The exam comprises one written paper in each of the following: I Biological Foundations & Cognitive Processes; II Individual Differences, Social & Developmental Psychology; III Research Design & Quantitive Methods in Psychology; IV General Paper; V Advanced Option Paper. A pass in the Qualifying Examination confers on the candidate eligibility for Graduate Membership of the Society and the Graduate Basis for Registration as a Chartered Psychologist.

Diploma in Clinical Psychology: Candidates must have the Graduate Basis for Registration as a Chartered Psychologist. British NHS trainee clinical psychologists are normally required to have completed three years of supervised service as trainees before being examined for the Diploma. Enquiries concerning other entry qualifications or other aspects of the exam should be addressed to the Registrar. The exam comprises: (a) one paper of three hours in each of the following: I Normal and Abnormal Development; II The Scientific Basis of Practice; III Change, Development and Innovation in Clinical Psychology; (b) five reports of clinical activity; (c) a small-scale research project; a research dissertation.

Diploma in Counselling Psychology: Candidates for the Diploma must hold the Graduate Basis for Registration of the BPS; they will normally be required to follow a three-year full-time or equivalent part-time path leading to the Diploma. The content of the Diploma comprises: (Part I) 150 hours of supervised counselling experience; experiential training workshops; a minimum of 40 hours of personal psychological counselling; submitted reports of counselling work; a three-hour written paper on the theory and practice of counselling; an interview at the discretion of the examiners; (Part II) 300 hours of counselling and 60 hours of supervision as a minimum; continuing experiential programme of skill development of a minimum 150 hours; submitted reports of counselling work; written paper on (a) psychology theory, clients and their concerns and (b) counselling process: research and outcomes; a dissertation of 4–5,000 words; two research projects of up to 8,000 words each; an oral exam.

Diploma in the Applied Psychology of Teaching: Candidates for the Diploma will normally be required to follow a two-year full-time or equivalent part-time path, leading to the Diploma, dated as from their enrolment. Before enrolment they must hold the Graduate Basis for Registration of the BPS and are normally required to have had four years' teaching experience under the guidance of a Chartered Psychologist who is a Teacher of Psychology. The exam comprises (1) four papers of three hours in each of (i) Cognitive Perspectives; (ii) Social & Personal Perspectives; (iii) Educational Perspectives;

(iv) Assessment; (2) Applied Teaching Assessment comprising: four case studies demonstrating the application of the theoretical material covered in Section A; six examples of the candidate's actual work on course structure and evaluation, eg samples of work assessed by the candidate; evidence of competence as a teacher from approved observers' reports on four occasions; a video recording of an actual teaching session; (3) an 8–10,000 word dissertation; (4) an oral examination at the discretion of the examiners.

Higher Degrees in Psychology Awarded by Universities

Because there are so many options taken with psychology, first degrees are not listed here. For full details, look at the *University and College Entrance Official Guide* or *British Qualifications*, both published annually.

Clinical Psychology

Applications to the courses listed below should be made through the Clearing House for Postgraduate Courses in Clinical Psychology, University of Leeds, 15 Hyde Terrace, Leeds LS2 9LT. Unless otherwise specified, all courses are 3 years full time.

Bangor: D.Clin.Psy
Belfast: MSc
Birmingham: Clin.Psy.D
East Anglia: Clin.Psy.D
East London: MSc
Edinburgh: MPhil
Exeter: Clin.Psy.D
Glasgow: M.App.Sc
Hull: BSc/Clin.Psy.D (6 yrs FT)(special psychology with clinical psychology)
Institute of Psychiatry, London: MSc
Lancashire: D.Clin.Psy
Leeds: D.Clin.Psychol or MSc
Leicester: MSc
Liverpool: M.Clin.Psychol
Manchester: MSc
Newcastle: MSc
North West Thames: MSc
Oxford: BPS qualification in clinical psychology
Plymouth: D.Clin.Psy
Sheffield: D.Clin.Psy
South East Thames: D.Clin.Psychol
Southampton: D.Clin.Psychol
Trinity College Dublin: MSc
University College Dublin: M.Psych.Sc (clinical specialisation) (2 yrs FT)

Educational Psychology

Belfast: MSc Developmental and Educational Psychology
Birmingham: MEd (Ed Psych.) Educational Psychology
Dundee: MSc Educational Psychology
East London: MSc Educational Psychology
Exeter: MEd Educational Psychology
Institute of Education, London: MSc Professional Educational Psychology
Manchester: MSc Educational Psychology

Newcastle: MSc Educational Psychology
Nottingham: MA/MSc Educational Psychology (professional training)
Sheffield: MSc Educational Psychology
Southampton: MSc and postgraduate certificate in Educational Psychology
Strathclyde: MSc Educational Psychology
Swansea: MEd Advanced study in Educational Psychology
Tavistock Clinic (Brunel University): MSc Educational Psychology
University College, London: MSc Educational Psychology

Occupational Psychology

Belfast: MSc Occupational Psychology
Bristol: MSc Organisational Psychology
Cardiff: MSc Occupational Psychology
East London: MSc Occupational and Organisational Psychology
Goldsmiths: MSc Occupational Psychology
Hertfordshire: MSc Occupational Psychology
Nottingham: MSc Occupational Psychology; MSc Occupational Psychology for British Students with GBR
Sheffield: MSc Occupational Psychology
Surrey: MSc Occupational and Organisational Psychology
UMIST: MSc Organisational Psychology

Psychotherapy

British Association of Psychotherapists, 37 Mapesbury Road, London NW2 4HJ. There are two parallel courses, one based on psychoanalytical (Freudian) and the other on analytical (Jungian) psychology. The Jungian Section was approved for Membership by the International Association for Analytical Psychology in 1986. The training lasts a *minimum* of four years from the commencement of theoretical training. The student should be in therapy with an approved therapist at least three times a week throughout the training and until qualification.

A Training in Child Psychotherapy was recognised by the Association of Child Psychotherapists in 1986; students can therefore expect to become eligible, upon qualification, for employment under the NHS. The training lasts a *minimum* of four years. Recently a Training in Adult Psychotherapy for Qualified Child Psychotherapists has been introduced. The training lasts a *minimum* of two years.

Both psychoanalytical psychotherapy and analytical psychology (Jungian) offer shorter external courses of particular interest to workers in the helping professions, who will have the opportunity to extend their understanding of a psychodynamic way of working in their day-to-day work. Full details of all these training courses can be obtained from the Secretary.

The Psychotherapy Centre, 1 Wythburn Place, London W1H 5WL.
The course is concerned with helping people who have emotional or psychogenic problems, enabling them to free themselves of these problems and function healthily. It is based on understanding relevant psychological, social and physiological factors. Prospective trainees, to gain insight and ensure that they are reasonably free of neuroses which could adversely affect their treatment of patients, first of all have extensive therapy with a practitioner designated for this purpose by The Psychotherapy Centre. The therapy, evolved in the light of 30 years of experience and long-term follow-up of results, is non-interpretative, non-suppressive, and free of indoctrination,

theory, religion or drugs. At the appropriate stage it is accompanied by lectures and practical work, including giving therapy under supervision and giving talks. The course, including therapy, normally takes at least four years full-time or part-time.

Applicants must have a university degree or equivalent. Some psychology graduates take the course as postgraduate training to help their clients adequately, but any degree is as relevant and acceptable; probably an arts degree is most suitable. A Diploma in Psychotherapy may be obtained. The course is to the standard of, and recognised by, the Psychotherapy Register.

Association of Child Psychotherapists, Burgh House, New End Square, London NW3 1LT. Members can be admitted to the Association after completing a postgraduate course of training recognised by the ACP and the DSS. The minimum requirements for entry into the four courses presently available are a degree and experience of working with young children. Details of these courses can be obtained from the Secretary of the ACP.

Higher Degrees

Central England: MSc Counselling and Psychotherapy
Kent: MA Psychotherapy
Leeds: MSc Psychotherapy
South Bank: MSc Psychotherapy/Psychosexual Therapy

Diplomas

Postgraduate Diplomas in Psychotherapy: courses at the Universities of Aberdeen, Liverpool, Sheffield and Warwick. Two to four years, full or part time, for candidates with registerable qualifications and suitable experience.

Psycho-Analysis

The British Psycho-analytical Society, 63 New Cavendish Street, London W1M 7RD, has Members and Associate Members who are elected after a qualifying training and who may describe themselves as 'psychoanalysts'. The Society is affiliated to the International Psycho-Analytical Association and its training organisation is the only one recognised by the International Psycho-Analytical Association as authorised to train psychoanalysts in the UK.

Training

Applicants for training are eligible for consideration if they are (a) medically qualified or undergoing medical training; (b) not medically qualified but have a good university degree, or its equivalent, and either have had relevant clinical experience or have, in the course of their professional work, carried other responsibilities for the development or welfare of individuals. The most appropriate disciplines would include social work, anthropology, psychology and sociology. The length of training varies, but the minimum is four years' part-time study. The training consists of (a) a personal psychoanalysis; (b) a three-year course of lectures and seminars requiring attendance on three evenings a week during term time; (c) psychoanalysis of patients under supervision; (d) other medical experience. Students, whether medically qualified or not, who have not had sufficient psychiatric experience in close clinical contact with patients, are required to obtain this. A training in the psychoanalysis of children and adolescents may be undertaken by qualified analysts and students nearing completion of the adult training.

Higher Degrees
The following are independent theoretical study courses and not clinical degree courses. They are run by universities and have nothing to do with training specified for potential psychoanalysts as outlined above.

Brunel: MA Psychoanalytic Studies
Essex: MA Psychoanalytic Studies
Guildhall: MA Psychoanalysis and Culture
Kent: MA Psychoanalytical Studies in the Humanities
Leeds: MSc Psychoanalytic Studies
Middlesex: MA Psychoanalysis
Sheffield: MA Psychoanalytic Studies

Counselling

British Association for Counselling (BAC), 1 Regent Place, Rugby, Warwickshire CV21 2PJ.
BAC membership is open to anyone counselling, using counselling skills within another role or training in counselling. The four categories of individual membership are: Associate, Full Individual, Approved and Fellow. Organisational Membership is also available.

Accreditation as an individual practising counsellor is awarded to individual members who successfully demonstrate that they meet one of the following criteria:

450 hours of completed formal counsellor training comprising 250 hours of theory and 200 hours of skills training, and at least 450 hours of supervised counselling practice over a minimum of three years; *or*
completion of a BAC recognised course plus supervised counselling practice as above; *or*
a ten-unit combination of counsellor training (one unit is the equivalent of 75 hours) and ten years of supervised practice (one unit is the equivalent of 150 hours minimum per year); *or*
ten years of supervised counselling practice with a minimum of 150 practice hours per year.

In all cases members must have an agreed on-going arrangement for counselling supervision of 1.5 hours or equivalent monthly and give evidence of serious commitment to on-going personal and professional development. This could be indicated by regular participation in further training, support study, personal therapy, etc.

Accreditation is awarded for five years only and must be reapplied for at the expiry of that period. Please apply to BAC for full details.

Degrees of Institutions of Higher Education

Higher Degrees
Birkbeck: MSc Psychodynamic Counselling
Bradford: MA Counselling in the Community
Bretton Hall College: MA Counselling
Bristol: MSc Counselling
City: Post MSc Practice of Counselling Psychology
College of Ripon and York St John: MA Counselling; MEd Counselling and the Management of Human Resources

Derby: MA Counselling; MEd Counselling, Personal and Professional Development
Durham: MA Counselling
East London: MSc Counselling Psychology
Goldsmiths College: MSc Counselling
Hertfordshire: MA Counselling
Hull: MSc Counselling
Keele: MA Counselling Studies; MA Counselling in Primary Care
Luton: MA Guidance and Counselling of Adults
Nottingham: MA Counselling Studies
Nottingham Trent: MA Counselling
Reading: MA Counselling
South Bank: MSc Careers Counselling and Guidance
Surrey: Counselling Psychology
Sussex: MA Counselling Psychology

Social Work

All social workers must take a course of professional training which usually contains an element of teaching about common psychiatric problems. Those who wish to specialise further may choose from a limited number of postgraduate courses.

Higher Degrees
Birmingham: MSocSc Social Work
Bradford: MA Social Work and Social Care
Bristol: MSW Social Work
Central England: MSc Health and Social Care
Dundee: MSW Social Work
Durham: MA Social Work
East London: MA Social Work Studies
Edinburgh: MSc Advanced Social Work Studies in Criminal Justice; MSW Social Work
Exeter: BPhil Social Work
Glasgow: MSW Social Work
Hertfordshire: Social Work Studies: Policy, Research and Evaluation
Keele: MA Social Work
Kent: MA Social Work; MA Social Work Studies
Kingston: MA Social Work
Lancashire: MA Social Work Studies
Manchester Metropolitan: MA Social Work; MA Social Work Studies
Manchester: MA Social Policy and Social Work
Reading: MA Social Work
Robert Gordon: MSc Applied Social Studies
South Bank: MSc Social Work
Southampton: MSc Social Work
Stirling: CCETSW Social Work Management
Sussex: MA Social Work; MA Social Work Studies
Warwick: MA Social Work
York: MA Social Policy and Social Work; MSW Social Work

Chapter 9

Useful Addresses

General

Universities and Colleges Admissions Service (UCAS), PO Box 67, Cheltenham, Gloucestershire GL50 3SF. (For applications to medical schools only, write to UCAS, c/o Fulton House, Jessop Avenue, Cheltenham, Gloucestershire GL50 3SH.)

The Educational Grants Advisory Service, c/o Family Welfare Association, 501–505 Kingsland Road, London E8 4AU; tel 0171 254 6251.

Medical

General Medical Council, 44 Hallam Street, London W1N 6AE; tel 0171 580 7642.

British Medical Association (BMA), BMA House, Tavistock Square, London WC1H 9JP; tel 0171 387 4499.

British Medical Association Education Trust, BMA House, Tavistock Square, London WC1H 9JP.

British Postgraduate Medical Federation, 33 Millman Street, London WC1N 3EJ.

Addresses of Regional Postgraduate Medical Deans

Northern region
Professor J Anderson FRCP FRCOG
Postgraduate Dean and Director
10–12 Framlington Place
Newcastle upon Tyne NE2 4AB

South Trent region
Professor John Walls
Postgraduate Dean
University of Leicester
Robert Kilpatrick Clinical Sciences Building
Leicester Royal Infirmary
PO Box 65
Leicester LE2 7LX

North West Thames region
Professor C S F Easmon
Regional Postgraduate Dean
BPMF
33 Millman Street
London WC1N 3EJ

South East Thames region
Dr M Cochrane
Postgraduate Dean
BPMF
33 Millman Street
London WC1N 3EJ

Wessex region
Dr H S Platt
Postgraduate Dean
Postgraduate Medical Centre
Highcroft
Romsey Road
Winchester SU22 5DH

North Western region
Professor I B Houston
Dean of Postgraduate Medical Studies
The University of Manchester Medical School
Stopford Building
Oxford Road
Manchester M13 9PT

Yorkshire region
Dr R Macdonald
Postgraduate Dean
PGME Department, West Wing
Yorkshire Health Buildings
Park Parade
Harrogate HG1 5AH

East Anglian region
Dr J Biggs
Regional Postgraduate Dean
University of Cambridge
School of Clinical Medicine
Addenbrooke's Hospital
PO Box 111
Hills Road
Cambridge CB2 2QQ

North East Thames Region
Dr J Tinker
Regional Postgraduate Dean
BPMF
33 Millman Street
London WC1N 3EJ

South West Thames Region
Dr H Seeley
Regional Postgraduate Dean
BPMF
33 Millman Street
London WC1N 3EJ

Oxford region
Dr W M G Tunbridge
Director of Postgraduate Education and Training
The Medical School Offices
John Radcliffe Hospital
Headington
Oxford OX3 9DU

West Midlands region
Professor J Temple
Dean of Postgraduate Medical and Dental Education
The Medical School
University of Birmingham
Birmingham B15 2TT

Mid Trent region
Dr R V Boyd
Postgraduate Dean
Medical School
Queen's Medical School
Nottingham NG7 2UH

North Trent region
Professor C L Welsh
Postgraduate Dean
University of Sheffield
Medical School
Beech Hill Road
Sheffield S10 2RX

Cardiff region
Professor T M Hayes FRCP
Dean of Postgraduate Studies
University of Wales, College of Medicine
Heath Park
Cardiff CF4 4XN

Co-ordinator for the regions
Dr Trevor J Bayley FRCP
Dean for Postgraduate Medical Education and Regional Adviser for Postgraduate Medical Education
Postgraduate Office
Faculty of Medicine
University of Liverpool
PO Box 147
Liverpool L69 3BX

Dentistry

British Dental Association, 64 Wimpole Street, London W1M 8AL; tel 0171 935 0875.

General Dental Council, 37 Wimpole Street, London W1M 8DQ; tel 0171 486 2171.

Addresses of Regional Postgraduate Dental Deans

England:

East Anglia region
G T Cheney
Regional Postgraduate Office
The Clinical School
Addenbrooke's Hospital
Hills Road
Cambridge CB2 2QQ

Mersey region
Dr J D Lilley
Dean of Postgraduate Dental Education
Fifth Floor
School of Dentistry
Pembroke
Liverpool L3 5PS

Northern region
D G Smith
Regional Postgraduate Institute for Medicine & Dentistry
10–12 Framlington Place
Newcastle upon Tyne NE2 4AB

North Western region
Miss G V Gilbe
Department of PG Medical & Dental Education
Dental School
Gateway House
Piccadilly South
Manchester M60 7LP

Oxford region
Dr J Rayne
Regional Director of Postgraduate Dental Education
Medical School Offices, Level 3
John Radcliffe Hospital
Headington
Oxford OX3 9DU

South Western region
D Seel
Dental Postgraduate Dean
Bristol Dental Hospital
Lower Maudlin Street
Bristol BS1 2LY

Thames region
D C Rule
Dean of Postgraduate Dentistry
British Postgraduate Medical Federation
33 Millman Street
London WC1N 3EJ

Trent region
Professor P S Rothwell
Regional Postgraduate Dental Dean
School of Clinical Dentistry
Wellesley Road
Sheffield S10 2SZ

West Midlands region
Professor J W Frame
Regional Postgraduate Adviser in Dentistry
The Dental School
The University of Birmingham
St Chad's Queensway
Birmingham B4 6NN

Yorkshire region
J P Ralph
Postgraduate Dental Dean
Level 6
Worsley Building
Clarendon Way
Leeds LS2 9LU

South and West Region
R T Reed
Postgraduate Dean's Department
Highcroft
Romsey Road
Winchester SO22 5DH

Scotland:

Grampian & Highland area
N W Kerr
Postgraduate Adviser in Dentistry
Department of Dental Specialties
Aberdeen Royal Infirmary
Aberdeen AB9 2ZB

Tayside area
F C McManus
Postgraduate Adviser in Dentistry
Dental School
Park Place
Dundee DD1 4HN

South-East Scotland
Mr Hew Mathewson
Postgraduate Dental Adviser for South East Scotland
11 Hill Square
Edinburgh EH8 9DR

West of Scotland
Dr J S Rennie
Postgraduate Adviser in Dentistry
West of Scotland Centre for Postgraduate Dental Education
378 Sauchiehall Street
Glasgow G2 3JZ

Wales:
E S Nash
Director of Postgraduate Dental Education for Wales
University of Wales College of Medicine, Room 155
Dental School
Heath Park
Cardiff CF4 4XY

Northern Ireland:
D H Saunders
Postgraduate Dental Tutor
Postgraduate Adviser in Dentistry
School of Dentistry
Grosvenor Road
Belfast BT12 6BE

Complementary Medicine

For general information contact the following two umbrella organisations:

Council for Complementary and Alternative Medicine, 179 Gloucester Place, London NW1 6DX; tel 0171 724 9103

Institute for Complementary Medicine, PO Box 194, London SE16 1QZ; tel 0171 237 5165

For information about the fields of complementary medicine mentioned in this book contact the following:

British Acupuncture Council, Park House, 206–208 Latimer Road, London W10 6XY

General Council and Register of Osteopaths, 56 London Street, Reading, Berkshire RG1 4SQ

National Association of Counsellors, Hypnotherapists and Psychotherapists, 145 Coleridge Road, Cambridge CB1 3PN

National Federation of Spiritual Healers, Old Manor Farm Studio, Church Street, Sunbury-on-Thames, Middlesex TW16 6RG

National Institute of Medical Herbalists, 56 Longbrook Street, Exeter, Devon EX4 6AH

National School of Hypnosis and Psychotherapy, 28 Finsbury Park Road, London N4 2JX

Society of Homoeopaths, 2 Artizan Road, Northampton NN1 4HU

Society of Teachers of the Alexander Technique, 20 London House, 266 Fulham Road, London SW10 9EL

Mental Health

Further information about training and job opportunities can be obtained from the following:

Association of Child Psychotherapists, Burgh House, New End Square, London NW3 1LT
Association of Cognitive Analytic Therapists, Munro Clinic, Guy's Hospital, London SE1 TRT
British Association for Counselling, 1 Regent Place, Rugby CV21 2PJ
British Association of Psychotherapists, 37 Mapesbury Road, London NW2 4HJ
British Psycho-Analytical Society, 63 New Cavendish Street, London W1M 7RD
British Psychological Society, 48 Princess Road East, Leicester LE1 7DR
Central Council for Education and Training in Social Work, Derbyshire House, St Chad's Street, London WC1H 8AE (Psychiatric Social Work)
Institute of Psycho-analysis, 63 New Cavendish Street, London W1M 7RD
Institute of Psychotherapy & Social Studies, 18 Laurier Road, London NW5 1SG
London Centre for Psychotherapy, 19 Fitzjohns Avenue, London NW3 5JY
MIND (National Association for Mental Health), Granta House, Broadway, London E15 4BQ
The Psychotherapy Centre, 1 Wythburn Place, London W1H 5WL
Society of Analytical Psychology, 1 Daleham Gardens, London NW3 5BY
United Kingdom Council for Psychotherapy, Regent's College, Inner Circle, Regent's Park, London NW1 4NS